Praise for
GIFTING KIDNEYS

"This book is a must-read for anyone considering living kidney donation, being evaluated for living kidney donation, or who has previously donated a kidney. Authors Tami Winchell and Laura Perin provide a comprehensive overview that includes both basic and in-depth information in an easy-to-read format. I was impressed by how well they describe the benefits as well as the risks of kidney donation and the practical advice they give. Their inclusion of stories from prior living donors is a highlight. I will recommend this book to all the living donor candidates that I meet with."

—**Michelle A. Josephson, MD**
President, **AMERICAN SOCIETY OF NEPHROLOGY**

"This book is an excellent tool for those considering living kidney donation. It clearly outlines the process, critical aspects to consider and understand, and shares the thoughtful, real-world experiences of those who have been through it. I wish our family would have had this book last year as a resource when my eldest son was going through the physical and emotional process of considering living kidney donation for his younger brother. In the end, he saved his brother's life, and they are both well. This book will help many others as they seek to make an informed choice about sharing the gift of life."

—**Lisa Bonebrake,** Alport syndrome patient and parent
Executive Director, **ALPORT SYNDROME FOUNDATION**

"I only wish I had a book like this when I was going through the transplant process. I'm so glad you were able to make something so important for donors!!!"

—**Elisa Schenkman,** Living Kidney Donor
Founder, **GOFARR FOUNDATION**

This book contains information relating to healthcare. It should be used to supplement, not replace, the advice of a trained health professional. The authors and publisher of this book provide the contents for information only and do not dispense medical advice or prescribe the use of any form of treatment for physical, emotional, or medical problems without the advice of a physician, either directly or indirectly. The publisher and the authors disclaim any liability, loss, or risk personal or otherwise, that is incurred as a consequence, directly or indirectly, of the use and application of any of the contents of this book.

Copyright©2023 by Tami WInchell. All rights reserved. Printed in the United Stated of America. No part of this book may be used or reproduced in any manner without written permission except in the case of brief quotations embodied in critical articles and reviews.

ISBN 979-8-9876379-1-3

Special discounts available for bulk sales.
For information: contact@giftingkidneys.com

FIRST EDITION

Cover Illustration by Gavin Winchell
Interior Illustrations by Astgik Petrosyan

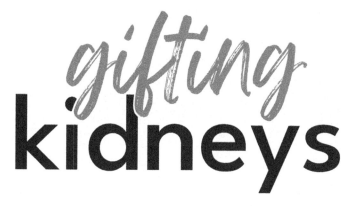

THE MASTER GUIDE TO LIVING KIDNEY DONATION

BY LIVING KIDNEY DONORS

TAMI WINCHELL, BCPA
with LAURA PERIN, PHD

Contents

INTRODUCTION • 1

CHAPTER ONE
What Are Kidneys? • 5

CHAPTER TWO
What Is Kidney Disease? • 11

CHAPTER THREE
How Is Kidney Failure Treated? • 25

CHAPTER FOUR
How Do I Become a Donor? • 33

CHAPTER FIVE
Who Can Donate to Whom? • 49

CHAPTER SIX
What Are the Health Risks of Donation? • 59

CHAPTER SEVEN
What Might I Expect From Surgery and Recovery? • 69

CHAPTER EIGHT
Will Donating Cost Financially? • 89

CHAPTER NINE
What Emotions Might I Expect to Feel? • 97

CHAPTER TEN
How Do I Stay Healthy With One Kidney? • 115

Donor Resources • 133
References and Additional Reading • 139
By Living Kidney Donors • 155

Introduction

Organ donation is the greatest of all gifts. One that has the power to grant others a renewed chance to not only survive, but to thrive, dream, and experience the fullness of life. It is truly amazing that, thanks to the tremendous generosity of organ donors, one million of these precious gifts have been transplanted in the United States alone.

Most are kidneys. The bean-shaped organ with a legume namesake.

Kidneys are vital to life, we cannot survive without them. Yet, one out of every seven Americans has diseased kidneys to some level.[1] This has led to a public health crisis, as kidney failure is one of the leading causes of death worldwide.[2,3] With the steeply rising rates of the two most common causes of chronic kidney disease, high blood pressure and diabetes, it is no surprise that kidney failure is also on the rise. These conditions account for three out of every four new kidney failure cases.[4]

When faced with kidney failure, lifetime replacement therapy, either dialysis or a kidney transplant, is required to survive. At present, there are 90,000 people on the national waitlist for a kidney transplant, with someone new added every 14 minutes—without a kidney available for them.[5] Most transplanted kidneys come from deceased donors, but the supply is simply not enough to match the demand. As a result, people often wait 3 to 5 years for a transplant, and even longer in some parts of the country.[6]

Without a transplant, people with failed kidneys must rely on dialysis to live. Dialysis is a life-prolonging treatment that filters blood but does not do everything kidneys do for us. As a result, those on dialysis are often unable to maintain normal lives[7] and their lifespan is typically shorter than those who receive a transplant. This is why about 17 people die every day while on dialysis and waiting for a kidney.[8] This is also why we see ads on social media and cars turned into billboards of those desperately seeking the gift of this vital organ.

With the rising kidney failure rate and the critical shortage of deceased donor organs, living donors have become increasingly crucial in this fight. Each year, about 6,000 healthy adults selflessly donate their kidneys to help family, friends, and even complete strangers.[9] However, despite their incredible gifts of kindness, the shortage remains.

More kidney donors are needed.

This is why living kidney donors created *Gifting Kidneys* to encourage informed and responsible donation and support those considering or undergoing the process. Donating a kidney is not always straightforward; the process can be pretty intimidating and complex. It can also be an emotional experience, with donors often feeling a wild ride of sentiments, from excitement and eagerness to fear and anxiousness. In fact, fear of the unknown may be the most unnerving aspect and could be a barrier to becoming a kidney donor for many. We understand all too well. We felt these emotions ourselves. It was not without hesitation or worry when we raised our hands to give our kidneys.

Through our own experiences and those of countless other donors, we have learned that being well-informed is instrumental in feeling confident in the choice to donate and ensuring the best possible experience. However, most in-depth donor education is only available after the commitment to undergo testing at a transplant center. Add to that, the sheer amount of information presented during a donor evaluation can be overwhelming and challenging to fully process. This can make the decision to donate tough or the decision to decline even tougher and emotionally charged, especially when a recipient is expecting a kidney.

Now, this compilation of information from respected transplant authorities featuring personal input from an array of multinational kidney donors is available to anyone at any time in the donation process. In a simple question-and-answer format, *Gifting Kidneys* answers all the commonly asked questions about kidneys and kidney disease, donor eligibility and the donation process, donor-recipient compatibility, the risks involved, financial and emotional aspects of donation, what to expect for the surgery and recovery, how to maintain good health with one kidney, and more. It empowers those thinking about kidney donation to make a fully informed decision and prepare for what comes next if they choose to gift the chance for renewed life to another. Whether readers consume *Gifting Kidneys* all at once, reference it as needed, or both, it provides valuable assistance, comfort, and advice at every stage of the donation process. By providing this information publicly, we can also help to normalize kidney donation and encourage healthy individuals to explore if giving this gift is right for them.

The need for kidney donors is both urgent and growing, as many suffering from kidney failure seek hope for a brighter future that only organ donation can provide. However, not everyone is a suitable candidate to donate a kidney. To help ensure the safety of both the donor and the kidney recipient, donor candidates must undergo a rigorous evaluation and approval process by a transplant center. Fortunately, for those who are not eligible to donate or decide that living donation is not right for them or not right for them at that time, there are still impactful ways to make a difference. For example, registering for deceased organ donation and encouraging others to do the same can lessen the demand for living donors. Raising awareness about kidney disease, prevention, and the need for living kidney donors are other powerful ways to join the mission to improve lives. At the end of the day, it is all about creating a better tomorrow for those who are struggling today or, even better, preventing them from struggling in the first place.

This highly informative guide is perfect for anyone curious about this extraordinary gift. It speaks intimately and directly to past and future donors, but it is also uniquely valuable for sharing with family and friends to foster support through the donation experience. Those who need a kidney donor will also find that this guide provides the information needed to feel comfortable and confident discussing this delicate topic with others and give them a straightforward resource to share with anyone expressing interest in exploring kidney donation further. Ultimately, this guide serves as a catalyst for open and informed communication, fosters empathy and understanding, and inspires hope for a brighter future.

Working together, we can make strides toward ending the needless loss of lives because of kidney disease. So please, share what you learn and become a *Gifting Kidneys Advocate*!

It is our honor to be on this journey with you.

—Tami Winchell, BCPA and Laura Perin, Ph.D.
Living Kidney Donors

CHAPTER ONE

What Are Kidneys?

Get ready to discover the superheroes of the body—the kidneys! These amazing organs are constantly working to keep us healthy and alive, yet people largely don't even know what they do.[10] Kidneys are best known for producing urine,[11] but they do so much more. In fact, they are incredibly complex organs connected to nearly everything the body does. That is why when the kidneys do not function well, almost every part of the body can be affected. By appreciating the significance of these unsung heroes, we can better understand the need for donating kidneys to those whose kidneys have failed. But you may wonder how we can donate a kidney when they are so essential to our health. Fortunately, although nearly everyone is born with two kidneys, it is possible to live a normal, healthy life with just one—as long as it functions well enough to do everything kidneys do for us sufficiently. Therefore, learning about these remarkable organs may inspire you to consider donating one of yours to someone whose kidneys can no longer keep them alive—and become a superhero yourself.

> At just 12 years old, my life was turned upside down when my kidneys failed due to the genetic disease Alport's syndrome. The journey that followed was filled with an immense health struggle. Until my dad, my hero, selflessly donated one of his kidneys to save my life. With his gift, I could achieve things I never thought possible. I have a great family life, graduated with

a master's degree, and am actively planning my future. Plus, my journey doesn't end there. My dad and I know how precious our kidney health is, and we make daily choices to protect it. I have made it my goal to set the record for the longest-surviving kidney transplant, a testament to the love and dedication that my dad has shown me. What's even more incredible is that my dad's selflessness has benefited him as well. Having one kidney motivates him to lead a healthier lifestyle, and he feels better than ever before. Donors can make an enormous difference in someone's life, just like my dad did for me. But first, I encourage those thinking about donating to get to know the kidneys and commit to a lifetime of kidney health."

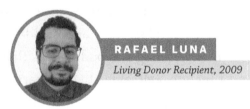

RAFAEL LUNA
Living Donor Recipient, 2009

Where are the kidneys and how do they work?

Nestled behind your belly sit two organs that look strikingly like overgrown kidney beans, one on each side of your spine. They're about the size of your fists but can vary depending on your body size and kidney health; they can shrink or enlarge when diseased.

Each kidney has about 500,000 to 1 million tiny parts, called *nephrons*,[12] responsible for the heavy work kidneys do. You can think of a nephron as a pool pump where water is sent through a filter to catch dirt and debris, and then the clean water is returned to the pool.

Each of these nephrons is made up of two parts: a *glomerulus* and a *tubule*. The glomerulus is a bundle of small blood vessels enclosed in a capsule serving as the filter to "clean" the blood. The tubule, surrounded by blood vessels, reabsorbs what the body needs to stay healthy and returns the filtered blood to the body. What's left is urine, the waste, which travels to the bladder through small tubes called ureters, one for each kidney. When the bladder is full, the urine exits the body through a tube called the urethra. Together, these parts make up the urinary tract—the kidneys, ureter, bladder, and urethra.

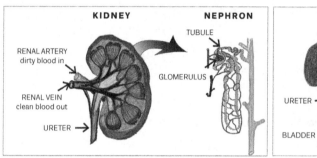
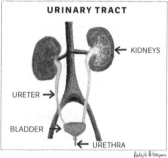

What do the kidneys do?

Have you ever really stopped to think about what your kidneys do? Kidneys play a major role in our health and survival, though they don't get much credit. According to a survey of 2,000 adults, the kidneys are generally not regarded as vital organs, like the heart or lungs, nor are they known for what they do. In fact, only half of those surveyed knew their most basic function, making urine.[13]

Despite their lack of recognition, our existence would not be possible without these hardworking organs. Kidneys are exceptional multitaskers that filter our blood, removing harmful toxins, chemicals, and other unwanted substances while also maintaining a healthy balance of fluids and electrolytes. At the same time, they are busy removing acids from the foods we eat, making hormones that control blood pressure, and activating vitamin D. And that's not all. Most people don't realize that kidneys also help keep bones strong and produce hormones that stimulate red blood cells to be made.[14] Kidneys are essential to life, as you can see, and deserve attention for all they do.

> **LEARN MORE**
>
> ## A Deeper Look Into What the Kidneys Do
>
> **Kidneys Purify Blood**
>
> Wastes are toxins, chemicals, excess food nutrients, and unwanted products created by body functions. Nephrons filter out these wastes from the bloodstream. If the kidneys do not have enough of them working as they should, wastes can accumulate in the blood to dangerous levels.
>
> **Kidneys Balance Fluids and Electrolytes**
>
> The amount of fluid and electrolytes circulating in the blood is balanced by the kidneys. Electrolytes are minerals such as calcium, phosphorus, sodium, potassium, and magnesium that we get from the foods and fluids we consume. The balance of these electrolytes helps keep us hydrated and are needed for proper cell, muscle, heart, brain, and nerve function.[15]
>
> **Kidneys Control Acidity**
>
> The foods you eat either increase or decrease the amount of acid in your body. When body fluids contain too much acid, problems result, such as muscle and bone loss, hormone problems, and kidney disease.[16] Keeping healthy levels of acid is an essential job for the kidneys. They do this by removing acid through urine.
>
> **Kidneys Make Hormones and Control Blood Pressure**
>
> Kidneys make hormones needed for many parts of the body to function.[17] One is vitamin D, which helps protect against disease and has many other vital roles. The kidneys must activate the vitamin D we get from food to become usable. Another is erythropoietin, which stimulates the bone marrow to make red blood cells that carry oxygen to the body's tissues. They also produce renin and angiotensin, which are needed to control blood pressure.

Kidneys Keep Bones Strong

Kidneys keep bones strong by maintaining the right balance of bone minerals and hormones.[18] These include phosphorus, calcium, vitamin D, and parathyroid hormone. Without enough kidney function, problems related to bone minerals and hormones can result. When extra phosphorus is not removed from the body, it can build up to damaging levels. As a result, vitamin D levels go down and too much parathyroid hormone is made. This causes calcium to move out of bones and into the blood, leaving bones weaker and more brittle.

Kidneys Clear Out Drugs

Along with the liver, kidneys work to clear medications and other drugs from the body. After a drug is taken, it travels through the bloodstream to the kidneys where the wastes are removed through the urine. Without good kidney function, drugs can build up in higher concentrations and cause serious problems.[19]

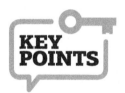

- Kidneys sit behind the belly, one on each side of the spine.
- Kidneys are vital for life; we cannot live without sufficient kidney function.
- Kidneys are much more important than we generally realize.

CHAPTER TWO

What Is Kidney Disease?

Think about this. Our kidneys filter about 150 quarts of blood every single day;[20] that's equivalent to a small bathtub filled to the brim. It's truly impressive when you consider the tiny size of their filters, the nephrons. Of course, unlike filters in cars or pools, we cannot simply replace our nephrons when they wear out and stop working. Instead, our filtering ability gradually declines over time with age; but this is usually not a problem since the kidneys can sufficiently do what is needed for us even with less filtering capacity. The real concern is when too much function is lost, such as when nephrons are consistently damaged by various factors you will soon learn about. Understanding the causes of nephron damage and how to detect problems early is important for helping to prevent some kidney diseases from occurring or for slowing their progression. What's more, knowing the causes can also empower us to advocate for awareness and prevention of chronic kidney disease.

What is nephrology?

It is reassuring to know that there are medical experts who specifically focus on diagnosing and treating kidney problems. These healthcare providers are called nephrologists. Other providers who manage kidney problems include primary care providers, pediatricians, urologists, and internists.

When learning about kidneys and talking to healthcare providers, you will sometimes hear the word *renal* and other times hear the word *kidney*. These words mean the same. *Renal function*, for example, means the same as *kidney function*.

What is a kidney injury?

Kidney injuries are when delicate nephrons are damaged, and they generally fall into one of two types: acute or chronic. Acute happens quickly and chronic happens gradually over time.

Acute Kidney Injury

You can think of an acute kidney injury as like a lightning strike, delivering a quick blow to the nephrons causing damage quickly. This type of injury may be caused by a range of factors, such as infections, physical injury, decreased blood flow, obstructions, and medications that are toxic to the kidneys.[21] Sometimes complete recovery is possible within a few weeks if the cause of damage resolves and treatment is received.[22] However, in more severe cases, dialysis may be needed temporarily to help the kidneys recover, and there may be a higher risk of developing chronic kidney disease in the future.[23,24]

Chronic Kidney Disease

Chronic kidney disease is different, more like a slow-burning fire, developing over months or years with progressively declining function.[25] Often, the goal of treatment is to slow down the progression rather than trying to reverse the damage. Unfortunately, chronic kidney disease is generally irreversible and typically worsens with time, although this is not always the case.[26]

What causes chronic kidney disease?

Whether you're an athlete or a couch potato, it is important to learn what causes damage to delicate nephrons, as kidney injuries can happen to anyone. By understanding what causes them harm and making choices that help them rather than hurt them, we improve their ability to do all they do for us throughout our lifetime.

The two most common causes of kidney failure are high blood sugar (diabetes) and high blood pressure (hypertension), which account for 60% to 70% of all failures.[27] Prevention or proper management of these conditions could eliminate most cases. Other causes of kidney injury leading to chronic kidney disease include inherited diseases, infections, autoimmune diseases, kidney stones, physical kidney injuries, obstructions, and dehydration. Certain lifestyle factors can also contribute to kidney damage, such as being overweight, having an unhealthy diet, smoking, and using certain nephrotoxic drugs. Taking steps to protect the kidneys by avoiding what causes kidney injury, where possible, reduces the risk of developing kidney disease.

> **LEARN MORE**
>
> ### Causes and Impacts of Kidney Injuries
>
> **High Blood Sugar**
> Too much sugar in the blood can damage many parts of the body, especially the kidneys, heart, blood vessels, and nerves. Diabetes is a condition that happens when the body does not produce enough insulin to keep up with the amount of sugar consumed. Type 1 diabetes typically begins in young people due to a pancreas that does not make enough, or any, insulin. Type 2 diabetes develops due to insulin resistance, generally caused by an unhealthy diet

and lack of exercise, and it is more common in overweight people.[28] About 1 in 3 adults with diabetes develop a kidney disease called diabetic nephropathy.[29] Over time, high blood sugar can damage nephrons and blood vessels, making them narrower and clogged. This restricts blood flow to the kidneys, causing nephrons to die, a loss of kidney function, and eventually potential kidney failure.[30]

High blood sugar can also harm nerves. If the nerves between the brain and bladder are damaged, the ability to feel when the bladder is full is lost. If the bladder becomes too full, urine can back up into the kidneys, causing extra pressure, which may damage their blood vessels. If the bladder is not emptied frequently enough, bacteria can grow in the urine and lead to a urinary tract infection. Left untreated, an infection may damage the kidneys. This is more likely to occur if the urine has high sugar levels.

High Blood Pressure

High blood pressure can damage blood vessels and result in chronic kidney disease. Healthy blood vessels are flexible and strong, with smooth inner walls that allow blood to flow freely. However, when blood pressure remains high over time, blood vessel walls become damaged and rough, causing fats from food to collect along the damaged surface and the walls to narrow and lose elasticity. This can affect the large arteries that go to each kidney and the tiny capillaries inside the nephrons. As a result, blood flow is impaired, and the nephrons cannot get the oxygen and nutrients they need to survive.[31] As more nephrons die, the kidneys' ability to filter fluid from the blood declines,[32] which can cause blood pressure to increase even more, creating a dangerous cycle.[33]

The causes of high blood pressure are like the causes of chronic kidney disease, such as genetic predisposition, being overweight, lack of physical activity, unhealthy diet, high blood sugar, stress, drinking too much alcohol, and smoking. Congenital conditions and other diseases can also contribute. Approximately half of the adults in the United States have high blood pressure[34] and it is also a risk factor for developing heart disease.

Heart Disease

Heart disease and kidney disease are directly related. Heart disease can cause kidney disease, and kidney disease can cause heart disease. Heart disease results from problems that keep the heart from pumping blood as it should, such as the buildup of plaque in the blood vessels, a blood clot, or a heart attack.[35] When the heart is not pumping blood efficiently, it becomes congested with blood, which increases pressure in the arteries that connect to the kidneys. This can clog the kidneys and prevent them from getting enough oxygen and nutrients to remain healthy.[36]

Inherited Diseases

Over 60 inherited diseases are known to affect the kidneys, ranging from common conditions to very rare.[37] While some inherited conditions may cause minimal problems, others may lead to kidney failure. Genetic testing can help to determine the chance of developing a genetic disorder and guide us in making informed decisions about our health. Genetic testing before living kidney donation is increasingly used to help evaluate donor candidate risks. A few inherited kidney conditions include the following.

- Polycystic kidney disease (PKD) causes cysts to grow in the kidneys which destroy their function.[38] It is the third most common cause of kidney failure.

- Alport syndrome is a condition that affects the collagen protein in the nephrons. Without healthy collagen, the blood vessels in the kidneys' glomeruli cannot function well.

- Fabry disease occurs when a gene that controls the body's ability to produce a specific enzyme, called alpha GLA, does not function right. This can affect the kidneys, heart, and nervous system.

Bacterial and Viral Infections

Bacterial and viral infections can damage kidneys directly by invading them or by causing other problems in the body that are harmful to the kidneys. These pathogens can enter the urinary tract through the urethra, the tube where urine is carried out of your body, and reach the kidneys.[39] They can also be carried to the kidneys through the blood from other parts of the body. For instance, hepatitis C and COVID-19 can travel to the kidneys and cause harm.[40] If not treated properly, kidney infections can cause permanent damage.

Autoimmune Diseases

An autoimmune disease is when the immune system malfunctions and attacks the body's own cells. Certain autoimmune diseases attack the kidneys, leading to inflammation, scarring, and damage to the nephrons.[41]

Obstructions

A urinary tract obstruction is a partial or complete blockage anywhere along the urinary tract. When urine cannot leave the body properly, it can cause kidney stones, infection, or cause urine to back up into the kidneys. If not treated, an obstruction can lead to loss of kidney function.[42]

Kidney Stones

Kidney stones are hard pebbles that form inside the kidneys due to factors like certain foods, specific medical conditions, excess weight, dehydration, various supplements, and some medications. They usually form in concentrated urine and can cause permanent kidney injury.

Excess Weight

Excess weight takes a toll not only on overall health but also contributes to kidney damage. The two leading causes of kidney disease—diabetes and high blood pressure—are often the result of excess weight. Furthermore, carrying extra weight forces the kidneys to work harder and filter more waste, increasing the likelihood of damage.

Diet
Eating an unhealthy diet high in inflammatory foods and low in nutritious foods increases the risk of kidney disease.[43] These foods can not only cause chronic inflammation that may directly damage the kidneys,[44] they can also lead to other risk factors that damage the kidneys, such as high blood sugar and high blood pressure.

Nephrotoxic Drugs
All drugs that enter the body must pass through the kidneys.[45] Though most medications and recreational drugs are metabolized in the liver, the kidneys are still responsible for eliminating their toxic waste products. It is important to know how some drugs can affect the kidneys, as nephrotoxic drugs are highly harmful and can cause kidney injury.

Smoking
Smoking is linked with a higher likelihood of developing kidney disease.[46] It may harm the kidneys in several ways, including increased heart rate and blood pressure, reduced blood flow, and narrowed blood vessels in the kidneys.[47]

Physical Injuries
Back muscles and the rib cage help protect the kidneys, but they can still become damaged from trauma. Blunt force trauma is one type of physical kidney injury, such as those obtained from sports, falls, and accidents. Another is penetrating trauma, such as those received from wounds or even medical treatments.

Dehydration
Dehydration happens when the body does not have enough fluid to function right. This is more likely after sweating heavily during

intense exercise, in hot climates, from uncontrolled diabetes, when sick, vomiting, or having diarrhea, and so on. When there's insufficient fluid is in the blood, the kidneys do not receive enough blood flow. This can cause a build-up of waste, acids, and can clog the kidneys. Severe dehydration or even mild dehydration over time can lead to kidney damage. [48]

Stress
The body's normal response to stress is the "fight or flight" reaction, which helps us cope with immediate dangers. During this response, heart rate increases, blood pressure spikes, muscles tense up, and levels of fats and sugars in the blood can rise. Stress experienced over an extended time can strain the kidneys and lead to kidney damage.[49]

What are the symptoms of kidney disease?

Kidney disease is a sneaky troublemaker that often goes undetected because it typically has no symptoms until the later stages. This is why it has earned the nickname, *the silent disease*. Shockingly, only 10% of those with kidney disease are even aware they have it.[50] Unfortunately, without symptoms, the kidneys may already be too damaged to save by the time kidney disease is diagnosed. Even when mild symptoms are present, they can easily be overlooked or attributed to other health issues. For instance, adults may simply feel tired and have less energy than usual. Early signs in young children may just include low weight or lack of growth.

Mild symptoms of kidney disease sometimes involve:[51]

- Less urine output
- Increased need to urinate

- Frothy urine
- Tiredness and less energy
- Trouble concentrating
- Difficulty sleeping
- Muscle cramping at night
- Dry, itchy skin
- Puffiness around the eyes, especially in the morning

In advanced stages of kidney disease, symptoms can become more intense, and new symptoms may appear, such as:[52]

- Making little or no urine
- Swelling of feet, ankles, hands, or face
- Shortness of breath
- Loss of appetite
- Stomach pain
- Loss of mental clarity or difficulty focusing
- Nausea or vomiting
- Weakness
- Blood in the urine

Routine blood and urine tests for kidney disease can help detect kidney problems before it is too late. When caught early, medical management may slow or stop the disease from getting worse.

How is kidney health tested?

Blood and urine tests are used initially to screen kidney health. If the results of these tests are not normal, it may indicate there is a problem, especially if they remain abnormal over time. In such cases, a healthcare provider may order additional tests, such as imaging or a biopsy, to confirm or rule out kidney disease.

LEARN MORE

Kidney Blood and Urine Tests Explained

BLOOD TESTS
Blood tests are critical for evaluating kidney health and for discovering problems early. Three primary blood tests used initially to measure kidney function include creatinine, glomerular filtration rate, and blood urea nitrogen.

Creatinine
Creatinine is a molecule that results from muscle use and digestion of dietary protein. It passes through the bloodstream and is filtered out of the body by the kidneys. Too much creatinine in the blood means there is not sufficient kidney function to filter creatinine at a normal rate. The higher the creatinine test result, the lower the filtration rate of the kidneys.

Glomerular Filtration Rate (GFR)
GFR measures the rate at which kidneys filter the blood. Complex testing is needed to accurately measure GFR, so an estimated GFR (eGFR) is often calculated instead using a formula that includes creatinine, age, sex, and body weight. As kidney function declines, GFR decreases. A GFR (or eGFR) result of under 60 (mL/min) for more than three months is generally considered chronic kidney disease.[53,54]

Blood Urea Nitrogen (BUN)
Blood urea nitrogen (BUN) is released when dietary protein is digested and can accumulate if the kidneys are unable to filter it. A high BUN result may signify that the kidneys are not functioning well.

URINE TESTS
Urine tests check for signs of kidney problems or other health conditions that affect the kidneys. Standard urine tests for kidney health include albumin, creatinine/creatinine clearance, and albumin to creatinine ratio.

Albumin

Albumin is a protein that should be in the blood, not the urine. Healthy kidneys do not let albumin pass into the urine. When albumin is found in the urine, it is called albuminuria or proteinuria. Three positive tests over three or more months signify a problem.[55] This can be one of the earlier signs of kidney disease.

Creatinine/Creatinine Clearance

A creatinine spot test detects creatinine in a single urine sample. The creatinine clearance test compares the creatinine in a 24-hour urine sample to the creatinine level in the blood. Both show how well the kidneys are filtering. The higher the result, the lower the filtration.

Albumin to Creatinine Ratio (ACR)

ACR is calculated by dividing the amount of albumin in the urine by the amount of creatinine. A higher result may indicate kidney disease.[56]

What are the stages of chronic kidney disease?

Chronic kidney disease progresses through stages based on how much kidney function is lost, which is determined using GFR. Depending on the stage of kidney disease, the goals of treatment differ. In the first three stages and early part of stage 4, the goal is to slow down the progression. But as the disease worsens, the risk of complications increases and additional management is needed. When the disease reaches advanced stage 4 and stage 5, dialysis or transplant is required.[57]

5 STAGES OF CHRONIC KIDNEY DISEASE		GFR = % OF KIDNEY FUNCTION
STAGE 1	Kidney damage with normal kidney function	90+
STAGE 2	Mild loss of kidney function	89-60
STAGE 3a	Mild to moderate loss of kidney function	59-45
STAGE 3b	Moderate to severe loss of kidney function	44-30
STAGE 4	Severe loss of kidney function	29-15
STAGE 5	Kidney failure	less than 15

What is stage 5 kidney failure?

Kidney failure is the daunting, irreversible loss of 85% to 90% of kidney function when the kidneys can no longer support the body. You may hear this critical state called stage 5 kidney disease or end-stage renal failure.[58,59] An unfortunate diagnosis of kidney failure occurs when GFR declines to less than 15.[60] At this level, another replacement therapy is required to stay alive, either dialysis or a transplant. When GFR reaches 20 or below, patients are eligible for a kidney transplant waitlist evaluation.

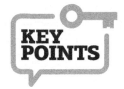

- Kidney disease means the tiny nephrons that filter blood are damaged.
- Slow and constant kidney injury causes most kidney disease cases over time.
- Simple blood and urine tests can detect if something is not normal with kidney function.
- The stages of chronic kidney disease are determined by how much kidney function has declined. Stage 5 is considered kidney failure and is not reversible.

CHAPTER THREE

How Is Kidney Failure Treated?

It's astonishing to think that nine out of ten people with kidney disease are unaware they have it.[61] Even more alarming is the fact that half of those with severe kidney disease, who are not receiving treatment, have no idea their kidneys are failing.[62] However, it is understandable why so many people don't realize they have kidney disease when you factor in the lack of symptoms and regular screenings, unmanaged underlying conditions, and limited healthcare access for some. Early diagnosis and management of kidney disease is crucial—before it reaches the point of no return.[63] While not possible in all cases, early intervention can often slow the progression of chronic kidney disease or even stop it from getting worse.[64] Progress has been made in raising public awareness of kidney disease and promoting early diagnosis and treatment, but more needs to be done as kidney failure continues to rise.[65] Not everyone with kidney disease will end up with kidney failure, but for those who do, replacement therapy is essential for survival—dialysis or a kidney transplant. Of those who need replacement therapy, about 70% are on dialysis, and 30% undergo a transplant.[66]

What is dialysis?

Dialysis is an impressive treatment that uses advanced technology to do some of the work kidneys normally do for us. It can be a lifesaving treatment that adds years to a patient's life for those waiting for a kidney, who cannot undergo transplantation, or who have rejected a transplanted kidney. With the help of a filtering machine or a special fluid in the belly, dialysis artificially "cleans" the blood and helps to control blood pressure.[67] Despite its benefits, however, dialysis cannot filter waste as effectively as healthy kidneys. It also cannot perform other work that kidneys do, such as making hormones.

Consequently, the average life expectancy on dialysis is 5 to 10 years, though some people have lived on dialysis for an incredible 20 to 30 years.[68] Moreover, dialysis is also very costly. The federal government pays a large portion, and health insurance helps, but people on dialysis may have to pay a costly portion too.

While dialysis can be lifesaving, living on dialysis can also be incredibly challenging. Patients spend many hours each week connected to the treatment at home or in a dialysis center. This limits their ability to work, travel, and spend time with friends and family. Spending time away from home requires careful arrangements to ensure continued treatments. Even eating and drinking are more complicated, with rigid diet restrictions required to avoid complications. And worse, troublesome physical symptoms of kidney failure and dialysis can make daily life tough.

As illustrated by dialysis nurse Linda Takvorian:

"Many children describe the sensation of dialysis as "like having bugs crawling under their skin." Children and adults tearfully describe unbearable leg cramps, abdominal cramps, chest pain, headaches, and body aches during the dialysis treatments followed by fatigue. Some adult patients start dialysis being able to walk unassisted to their dialysis chair. As the dialysis years pass, their bones and muscles waste at an accelerated rate. They eventually need assistance – a cane, a wheelchair, or a caretaker too early in their life. Some patients are hospitalized with renal fractures. Older patients are victims of "dialysis-related" complications that lead to multiple hospitalizations related to infections, cardiac events, or access failure. We care for our patients like they are our precious family and pray for transplants. Nurses understand the progression of renal disease and the importance of early transplant. Transplanted patients are delighted when they return to a normal lifestyle. Early transplant gives these patients a second chance in life. They gain back their lives and dreams."

 I could not live with the idea that my wife would spend so many years on dialysis."

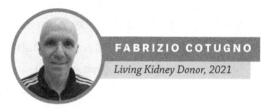

FABRIZIO COTUGNO
Living Kidney Donor, 2021

What is a kidney transplant?

A kidney transplant is an extraordinary medical procedure that involves surgically placing a healthy kidney from a living or deceased donor into someone whose kidneys have failed. This impressive treatment allows a single healthy kidney to do the work that two diseased kidneys can no longer do.

The benefits of a kidney transplant are profound. Successful transplants have the ability to extend a recipient's lifespan, restore their health, and make a better quality of life possible. With a healthy kidney taking care of the vital functions kidneys do for the body, recipients may return to everyday life without the challenges of dialysis treatments and difficult symptoms, enjoy more energy, and may engage in their work and personal life fully.

Beyond the physical benefits, a transplant can also positively transform emotional well-being. With it comes a renewed sense of hope and vitality, alleviating the anxiety and fear of failing kidneys and allowing recipients to confidently plan for their future. Furthermore, the advantages of restored health reach well beyond the recipient, touching the lives of loved ones and even those more distantly connected.

> "Expressing the significance of a kidney transplant is a challenge because it is a second chance at life for sure, but it is so much more. Its effects impact many more lives than just my own. As a husband, the transplant saved my wife's life. As a father, the transplant holds immeasurable significance for future generations. As an active community member, congregational leader, and business owner, the transplant touches lives far and wide. While the gift of a transplant may mean life and death to me, the impact on others is limitless. The influence of a kidney donation goes far beyond what is initially considered."
>
>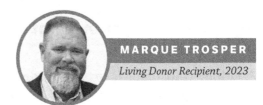
> **MARQUE TROSPER**
> *Living Donor Recipient, 2023*

Is a kidney transplant a cure?

Although kidney transplants can improve the health and prolong the life of a recipient, donors should recognize and accept that this outcome is not guaranteed. Complications and risks associated with the procedure and the medications used to prevent organ rejection can result in negative consequences. One such consequence is the significantly increased vulnerability to infections and cancer due to immune suppression.[69]

> " I donated to my spouse, but if I could turn back time, I would not do it. He has had nothing but complications since the transplant. You have to be willing and ready for anything that comes and realize that not all recipients have the outcome you desire for them."

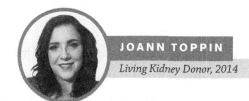

JOANN TOPPIN
Living Kidney Donor, 2014

Furthermore, donors should understand that kidney transplants treat kidney failure but are not always a cure. Those with certain genetic diseases that caused their kidneys to fail, such as polycystic kidney disease, will still have the disease, but the transplanted kidney will remain free of the disease. However, those with kidneys that fail due to certain diseases such as diabetes, obesity, lupus, or heart disease will still have these diseases after a transplant, and they must be managed effectively to prevent them from causing the transplanted kidney to fail.

What are the benefits of living kidney versus deceased kidney donation?

Living and deceased donor kidneys may equally improve the quality and length of life for a recipient. It's worth noting, however, that living kidney donation may provide some additional benefits to the recipient,[70] such as:

- Living donor kidneys may last longer.
- Living donation may shorten the wait time for a kidney transplant, which may help avoid health problems that dialysis can cause over time.

- Living donation may allow the recipient to receive a transplant preemptively before dialysis is required.
- Living donation may provide better genetic matches between the donor and recipient, which may decrease the risk of organ rejection.
- Living donation surgical scheduling is more practical.
- Living donation makes chain and paired exchange possible, giving more recipients a chance for transplantation.[71]

> "Donating my kidney was a feeling of elation and euphoria that is hard to put into words. I felt so happy for my kidney recipient."

COLLEEN FLANARY
Living Kidney Donor, 2018

How long do transplanted kidneys last?

Most kidney transplants are successful, giving recipients many years, or even a lifetime, with their new kidneys and renewed health. Sometimes, however, recipients may need more than one. The longevity differs from person to person.[72] Factors that may determine how long a transplanted kidney lasts include:

- The overall health of the recipient.
- Medical management of the recipient after the transplant.
- How well the kidney is matched.
- Time on dialysis prior to transplant.
- Taking immunosuppression medications as directed.
- Whether the transplanted kidney was from a living donor or deceased donor.

HOW IS KIDNEY FAILURE TREATED?

- Delayed kidney function after transplantation.
- The recipient's lifestyle habits.
- Whether kidney disease risk factors are well managed.
- Complications of immunosuppression medications.[73,74,75]

LIVING DONOR VERSUS DECEASED DONOR KIDNEY SURVIVAL RATES		
	Deceased Donor Kidney	Living Donor Kidney
Average organ survival[76]	8-12 years	12-20 years
1-year organ survival[77]	93%	97%
5-year organ survival[78]	78%	88%
10-year organ survival[79]	50%	66%

> " I donated to my father. It changed his life and brought him back to a wonderful state of health, so he was able to travel and enjoy life again. The truth is though that it changed my life too. It gave me such an incredible sense of pride and purpose. After giving my dad my kidney, I felt that even if I accomplished nothing more in my life of importance, my life now had value and purpose. I know it wasn't easy for him to take my kidney, pretty scary for a dad to take his child's healthy organ, but I would have given it to him 100 times over to give him those extra 12 years. Those extra twelve years allowed him to walk both my sister and me down the aisle for our wedding, allowed him to meet and get to know six more grandchildren, allowed him that time to travel and enjoy his life, and allowed me to get to know him through the eyes of an adult."

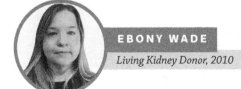

EBONY WADE
Living Kidney Donor, 2010

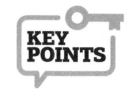

- The best treatment for kidney disease is early diagnosis and management—before it is too late.

- Nine out of ten adults with kidney disease are unaware they have it due to a lack of screening and symptoms.

- When faced with kidney failure, dialysis or a transplanted kidney is required to survive.

- Transplantation is the preferred treatment over dialysis, giving recipients the opportunity for a longer and better quality of life.

CHAPTER FOUR

How Do I Become a Donor?

It is fascinating that most of us are born with two kidneys, yet we can live a healthy life with just one, provided that it functions adequately enough to do all that kidneys do. This means that any healthy adult can potentially gift a kidney to someone whose kidneys are not working. First, however, anyone considering this generous gift must undergo a complete evaluation before being approved to donate. This evaluation is important for both the donor and the recipient to determine how the donation might affect the donor and if they have a kidney that is suitable for a recipient. The purpose of the evaluation is to minimize the risk for negative consequences.

While there are some risks of living donation, the thorough evaluation process provides a systematic way of minimizing these risks by looking at factors specific to the individual. About half of those who complete a full donor evaluation get approved. The frequency of acceptance varies with each transplant center and partly depends on specific eligibility standards.[80]

A living donor healthcare team at a transplant center completes donor evaluations. This team is assigned only to the donor and is not part of the recipient's healthcare team. This arrangement helps to ensure that there are no conflicts of interest. A living donor advocate is an important member of this team who is available for questions throughout the evaluation process and is there to ensure that donor rights are protected, respected, and maintained.

While the exhaustive evaluation is lengthy and sometimes

overwhelms donors, they typically regard the experience as very valuable for minimizing risks, becoming informed, and preparing for donation.

> The screening process is extensive. The testing, prep, and recovery isn't easy. It's hard to be a donor physically and psychologically. But, it will be the grandest thing you'll ever do."

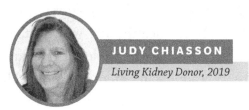

JUDY CHIASSON
Living Kidney Donor, 2019

Who can be a donor?

Approval from a transplant center after a careful assessment is required to donate. Although there are universal standards to promote consistency and safety, each center may interpret some guidelines differently and apply additional criteria. Every candidate is evaluated individually, but the basic guidelines include the following:

- At least 18 years or older
- Good overall health
- Two well-functioning kidneys
- A willingness to donate
- No history of high blood pressure that is difficult to control, kidney disease, diabetes, certain cancers, or major risk factors for heart disease
- Not excessively overweight (BMI over 35)
- No active drug or alcohol abuse
- Be willing to quit smoking before surgery
- No serious infectious diseases that could be passed to the recip-

ient, such as hepatitis C or HIV, unless approved to donate to a recipient with the same diseases

> I am so aware of my privilege to have good health and I know that donating my kidney was far easier than the health journey of a kidney recipient. Kidney donation is one of the most important things I have done in my life. I am so grateful to have had the experience."

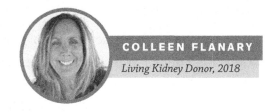

COLLEEN FLANARY
Living Kidney Donor, 2018

Am I too old to donate?

There is no specific age cutoff for donating a kidney, provided you are in good health and meet all criteria for donation. However, if you are an older donor, you may be paired with a more similarly aged recipient. It is important to note that age is just one factor, and the decision as to whether you are too old is based on many factors for you and your recipient.

> For my husband and me both at age 70, the doctors were less concerned about looking for a younger organ. Instead, they were looking at life expectancy for both of us to ensure my donation fulfilled both our needs—my single kidney could serve me for the rest of my life and my donated kidney could serve him through his remaining years. This is all that was needed and all we really wanted."

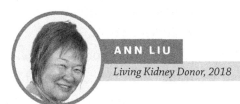

ANN LIU
Living Kidney Donor, 2018

How do I begin the donation process?

Getting the donation process started is slightly different depending on whether or not you have a specific person in mind to whom you would like to donate.

Directed Donation

If you already have someone in mind to whom you would like to donate, contact the transplant center where they are registered. While it is sometimes preferred that the donor and recipient have the surgery at the same center, if not feasible, donors may have the option to choose their own transplant center and have the organ transported to the recipient's location. In either case, the donor should contact the intended recipient's transplant center to begin the process.

Nondirected Donation

If you wish to donate your kidney but don't have a specific recipient in mind, you have two options. You can choose a transplant center to coordinate your gift with someone in need, or you can start by contacting the National Kidney Registry to get help with the living donor process.

How do I choose a transplant center?

In the event you are a nondirected donor or choose not to donate at your recipient's transplant center, consider the following factors when selecting your own.

It may be best to choose a center that is a preferred provider on your insurance plan. A recipient's insurance is responsible for the expenses directly related to the evaluation, the surgery, and the recovery, but sometimes other costs come up that are your responsibility. For example, the recipient's insurance may not cover additional tests or treatments that are required but not directly related to the donation, such as preventative screenings.

If you do not have a recipient, find out if the transplant center you are considering participates in paired or chain exchange programs. These programs can help you donate when you do not know someone who needs a kidney. In addition, if your transplant center is partnered with the National Kidney Registry (NKR), you may be eligible for additional benefits. Potential benefits include insurance protection during the donation phase, guaranteed life and disability insurance, legal support if terminated from your job for donating, and the option for an evaluation performed at an NKR-affiliated transplant center nearest your home. A list of participating centers is available from the National Kidney Registry at kidneytransplantcenters.org.

Keep in mind that not all transplant centers have the same outcomes. Therefore, it is smart to research how many living donor transplants the center performs each year, the frequency of complications, and the organ survival rates for kidney recipients. This information is available from the Scientific Registry of Transplant Recipients at srtr.org.

What happens when I first contact a transplant center?

Contacting a transplant center can feel a little intimidating if you don't know what to expect. But really, they keep the process of getting started straightforward and simple. The first step is an initial screening, which typically takes place with a phone call or online questionnaire. You'll be asked questions about your general health status and other qualifying factors. This determines if there are any obvious medical conditions or other criteria that may prevent you from donating.

Based on the results, if you are a nondirected donor, you may be invited to begin a donor evaluation. If you wish to donate to a specific recipient, you will need to provide a blood sample for compatibility testing. If after the initial screening you are considered a compatible candidate, approval to begin the donor evaluation may be given. If you don't live near the transplant center, alternatives for completing tests may be an option.

It's not uncommon for these initial encounters to feel impersonal with an unexpected lack of enthusiasm that doesn't match the grander of the donor offering. If this is your experience, just know that sometimes centers are working through volumes of donor candidates and regardless of these impersonal initial steps, you will be well cared for as you proceed through the process.

What is a donor evaluation?

A donor evaluation is an extensive series of tests and interviews to determine your eligibility to donate and minimize risks for you and the recipient. The evaluation focuses on three key areas: medical, financial, and psychosocial.[81]

Medical

The medical evaluation is a critical step in determining if you are eligible to donate. The goal is to make sure that your kidneys are healthy and viable for transplant and that you are in good overall health to donate safely. Extensive testing helps reduce the risk of any issues occurring from the surgery or in the future. While it may not be possible to test for all potential problems and future risks, the team will do their utmost to protect you.

This thorough evaluation will include an assessment of your health history, physical exams, and a battery of tests. These tests will look at your kidney function, past exposure to infectious diseases, cardiovascular and lung health, diabetes, cancer, and other relevant health concerns. Genetic testing is becoming more common in the evaluation to further identify any potential health risks that you may be prone to developing in the future. Additionally, you may be required to do prevention screenings, such as a mammogram, colonoscopy, and pelvic or prostate exam. And if an area of concern is found, additional tests may be required. There are many testing possibilities, and some are selected on a case-by-case basis.

Throughout the evaluation, your team will provide detailed information about the surgical procedure, potential risks, and after-surgery care. You will have many opportunities to ask questions and be carefully supported throughout the process.

COMMON DONOR EVALUATION TESTS

PURPOSE	TEST
Compatibility	ABO blood type verification
	HLA tissue typing
	Serum Crossmatch
Kidney Function	24-hour urine collection
	GFR measurement
	Urinalysis
	Ultrasound
Kidney Anatomy	CT or MRI
	Arteriogram
Glucose Intolerance	Fasting glucose
	Oral glucose tolerance
	Hemoglobin A1C
Hematological System	Blood tests
Cardiovascular	Lipid blood panel
	Blood pressure clinic readings
	24-hour BP monitoring
	Electrocardiogram (EKG)
Liver Function	Blood tests
Transmissible Infection	Venereal diseases blood tests
	Past or present viral screening
Cancer Risk	Cancer screening
	Family history evaluation
Lungs	chest x-ray

> "I was thoroughly supported throughout the comprehensive screening process. The medical team reviewed every test to ensure that I was healthy, well-informed, and comfortable enough to continue. It was the most thorough physical exam of my life. Learning just how healthy I was at age 65 was an unexpected bonus."

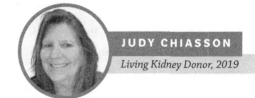

JUDY CHIASSON
Living Kidney Donor, 2019

Financial

All medical expenses related to the transplant should be covered by your recipient's insurance. However, other costs, such as lost wages, travel expenses, or medical care after donation, are not covered. These expenses can add up, but you don't have to navigate this alone. Your healthcare team will perform a financial evaluation to ensure your gift doesn't put you in a tough spot and to help you find aid if needed. To learn about the financial details of kidney donation, refer to Chapter 7.

Psychosocial

Protecting your mental health and ensuring you understand all aspects of living donation to make an informed decision is an important part of the evaluation. It involves assessing whether you acknowledge and voluntarily accept the risks and giving you private time with a transplant professional to express any concerns you might not feel comfortable sharing with family or the recipient present. For details about the psychosocial evaluation and the emotional factors of donation, see Chapter 9.

> "There is no greater gift than giving life to your child a second time. Our family was truly blessed that I was a kidney match for our 15-year-old son. Even though I'm his mother, I still had to go through all the physical and psychological tests to make sure that I was the best match. Honestly, I didn't think about risks to me because all I wanted was for my son to have a bright, healthy future. If I had more kidneys to give, I would definitely go through the process again. Is the process easy... no, but to save a person's life, you'll do anything."

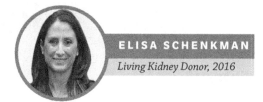

ELISA SCHENKMAN
Living Kidney Donor, 2016

Will my evaluation results be kept private?

Your medical record may not be shared with anyone unless you give permission, according to the Health Insurance Portability and Accountability Act (HIPAA). Therefore, your healthcare team may only notify the recipient that an evaluation is in progress and whether you have been approved to donate.

How long is the evaluation process?

The evaluation process takes time and can require some patience. Testing days are often long, and the tests can be uncomfortable. Sometimes the entire evaluation process takes weeks, and sometimes it can take many months. On average, you can expect anywhere from one to six months, but it may even go longer. Each transplant center has its own estimated time frame, depending on many factors, such as availability for scheduling tests, appointments, and specific evaluation policies. Moreover, each evaluation is unique and will vary with any additional testing needed for concerns.

Work with your donor team, follow through with their requests, and stay engaged with your donor advocate for the most timely and efficient evaluation process. A surgery date will not be set until the evaluation is complete and you are approved to donate.

> " The evaluation process went quick for me which I really appreciated. I do not like things drawn out. The waiting is the hardest for me. I do not like needles, blood, or surgery in general so that was not easy, but knowing the why of the process helped me get through it."

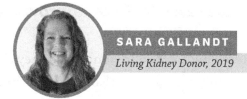

SARA GALLANDT
Living Kidney Donor, 2019

Candidates are evaluated to determine their eligibility based on what is best for their well-being. Certain conditions may result in a denial, but this is not always the case. The severity of certain conditions is also taken into consideration.

The following are general concerns that can prompt a denial. If any apply to you, talk to a transplant center for more information about your case.

- Kidney disease or strong family history of kidney disease
- Diabetes or strong family history of diabetes
- Significant obesity
- Positive HIV status (positive donors may only donate to positive recipients)
- A history of hepatitis (positive donors may only donate to positive recipients)
- Uncontrolled or newly diagnosed high blood pressure or the use

of multiple medications to control high blood pressure
- A history of more than one episode of kidney stones
- Chronic use of some medications for arthritis or other chronic pain
- Active cancer
- Uncontrolled mental illness
- Smoking (if unwilling to stop)
- Active drug and alcohol abuse
- Potential for financial hardship

What can I do if not approved to donate?

Receiving a denial to donate a kidney can be a devastating experience not only for you but also for the recipient and their loved ones who may have been counting on you. It can be disheartening to learn that despite your willingness to donate, you are not approved. However, there may still be options. As an example, your medical team may provide guidance to help you enhance your health and fulfill requirements that caused your decline for donation, such as weight and cardiovascular health. If these requirements as met, they may allow you to be reassessed. Other conditions, on the other hand, may cause a permanent denial, such as kidneys with evidence of disease. In this case, re-evaluation is not possible.

Complex emotions are normal and understandable if not approved, especially if your intended recipient is suffering and out of options. If this is your experience, consider reaching out for professional support to help avoid any negative impact on your emotional well-being if left unaddressed.

Keep in mind that if denied for living kidney donation, this does not mean you cannot donate a kidney or help those in need. Organ donation after death can be possible for many candidates who have been denied, and it's a critical need. Go to RegisterMe.org and make your wish known. You can also advocate for your intended recipient by spreading the word about their need for a kidney. Further, you can help by raising awareness for kidney disease, prevention, and the need for deceased organ donation and living kidney donors.

Who decides if I may donate?

Your evaluation will be meticulously reviewed by a highly experienced transplant team, which may include surgeons, nephrologists, psychologists, and social workers. The wait for their decision can be hard, with feelings of excitement, hope, and anxiety all intertwined. It's understandable to want a quick decision, but it often takes about two weeks and can take even more time.

Ultimately, the final decision of whether you donate a kidney or not is yours and must be both *informed* and *voluntary*.[82]

Informed

Education is a requirement of the donor process. It helps to ensure that you know the essential information necessary to make a knowledgeable decision about donating. If you are informed, you will understand:

- The donation process, including the surgery and recovery.
- The risks and benefits of donation.
- Your potential recipient has options for other treatments, including dialysis or a transplant from someone else.[83]

Voluntary

Your decision to donate must be based entirely on your own will, without pressure or bribery. If your decision is voluntary, you:

- Will not feel pressure to donate from anyone.
- Will know that you may decide not to donate at any time.
- Will not take a bribe or anything of monetary value for your donation.[84]

When approved to move forward with organ donation, it becomes your decision entirely. It is normal to feel a range of emotions at this point, such as excitement, uncertainty, guilt, or fear. Sometimes people are eager to donate before they fully understand the process and potential risks, resulting in pressure to go ahead with their gift even when they feel uncertain. If you need help making your decision, you can talk to your family or close friends, but it may be more comfortable and productive to speak with someone at the transplant center or other donors who have already gone through this experience.

Can I change my decision to donate?

Whether to donate or not will always be respected and honored by your transplant team. Throughout the process, members of the team will repeatedly ask if you wish to withdraw your offer confidentially. Changing your mind or needing more time is perfectly acceptable, and your team is there to help. If at any point you choose to delay or stop your donation for any reason, your donor advocate and the team will be there to support you and help you to decline in a way that protects your privacy and preserves your relationship with the recipient. According to your rights under HIPAA, the team may not disclose any of your personal information, including your reasons for terminating your donor candidacy. Your recipient will only be informed that you have been excluded from donating, and no one will be given any other information.

> " I did my research, asked questions, and trusted my transplant center. They are required to give you an out and they will not take your kidney if there are any signs of coercion or pressure. No one will force you to do it—you won't be trapped."
>
> **TRACEY BRADFORD**
> *Living Kidney Donor, 2022*

How long after approval is the surgery scheduled?

No predetermined timeframe exists for when the surgery will be scheduled after a donor is approved, which can make the waiting process difficult. If the surgery is scheduled six months after the initial approval, blood tests may need to be repeated. However, in most cases, donor evaluations are generally considered valid for one year. Sometimes scheduling is quick, within weeks, and sometimes it takes many months. Scheduling a transplant surgery depends on many factors, including the health of the recipient and the availability of the transplant center and team. It is not uncommon for scheduled surgery dates to be delayed when a recipient's health changes and it is determined that it is best to wait.

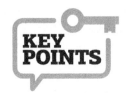

- Donor evaluations help to protect donor candidates from undue harm and to find out if they have a viable kidney for donation.
- Medical, financial, and psychosocial assessments are requirements of the donor evaluation.
- It can take anywhere from one to six months or more to complete the evaluation process.
- A donor candidate may opt out of donation at any time.

CHAPTER FIVE

Who Can Donate to Whom?

Kidney transplantation is a fascinating field that has seen incredible progress since the first successful living kidney donor transplant in 1954. In the early days, most donors were limited to biological relatives. But with advances in medicine and improved transplant treatment, successful transplants from less compatible donors are now possible. This means that today, extended family, friends, co-workers, and even strangers can be considered viable donor candidates, making many more transplants possible.

In the effort to further expand the number of transplants that can be performed, exchange programs have been established in recent years to organize trades between incompatible donor and recipient pairs. These arrangements are becoming increasingly common, making it possible for many more people to receive living donor kidneys. It is exciting to see the rise in lives saved thanks to these developments and to anticipate how further improvements will continue to be made in this evolving field.

While compatibility is no longer the major obstacle it once was, careful matching is still a crucial factor ensuring the best possible chance of a successful transplant.

Why is compatibility important?

You know compatibility is important to reduce the risk of rejection, but you may wonder why. Put simply, it's because we are all one of a kind—a recipe of unique cells, tissues, and organs—that our immune system knows very well and will destroy anything that does not belong to keep us safe. When transplanted, the immune system can see a donor organ as foreign and produce antibodies to attack it. Compatibility testing helps prevent this scenario. The more similarly matched a donor and recipient are, the more likely the recipient's immune system will not tag the organ as a threat.[85]

To help prevent the recipient's immune system from attacking the new organ, medications, called immunosuppressants, are taken for the lifetime of the transplanted organ to help keep it alive. However, they can only do so much. This is where compatibility comes in—it remains a necessity.

Although most kidney transplants are successful, there are times when the kidney is rejected. Hyperacute rejection, which can happen immediately after transplantation, is extremely rare due to advanced compatibility testing. Acute rejection can happen within the first year and affects about 10% to 15% of adult kidney recipients.[86,87,88] Chronic rejection, an ongoing attack, is not uncommon but can typically be controlled if detected early.

Exciting new medical advances are presently ongoing that will continue to improve the success of transplants and expand donor compatibility even further.

> " I knew immediately that kidney donation was for me. It just felt right. I had always thought about doing something like this, I was turning 60, and the opportunity came to me by chance through a conversation at work. Everything just fit together and I knew I was meant to donate."

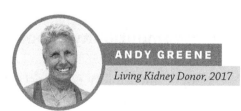

ANDY GREENE
Living Kidney Donor, 2017

How can I find out if I am a match?

Donor compatibility testing typically starts with a blood test to determine the blood type of both the donor and recipient. This is important because blood type compatibility is generally required for a successful transplant. If the blood types are compatible, then further tests are performed to check for tissue compatibility. This involves a series of tests that evaluate the recipient's immune system response to the donor's tissue. The results help determine the best donor match for the recipient.

About **1 in 3** donor candidates are not compatible with their intended recipient.[89]

LEARN MORE

Standard Compatibility Tests Explained

Blood Typing
Blood typing determines if a donor's blood type is suitable for a recipient. The compatibility of blood types is essential because some blood types have antibodies that can attack others leading to rejection of a transplanted organ. There are four blood types: O, A, B, and AB. The Rh factor (+ or -) does not affect compatibility. Some blood types are compatible with other blood types, but not all of them. In some cases where blood types are incompatible, a process called plasmapheresis may be an option to make a transplant still possible.

Human Leukocyte Antigen (HLA) Typing

HLA typing, also called tissue typing, compares the genetic antigen similarities between the donor candidate and recipient to determine the likelihood of organ rejection. Six antigens out of over 100 are important for organ transplantation. A test result of zero indicates no match, while a test result of six indicates an exact match. HLA types are inherited, so blood relatives are more likely to have a higher antigen match, with parents and children having at least a 50% chance and siblings with the same parents having a 25% chance. Unrelated donors are less likely to match. While a closer antigen match increases the likelihood of a successful transplant,[90] medications and desensitization strategies make transplants possible with less compatible HLA types.

Serum Crossmatch

A serum crossmatch is used to determined blood compatibility. During the test, the recipient's serum carrying antibodies is mixed with white blood cells from the donor. A positive crossmatch occurs if the recipient's antibodies attack the donor's cells, meaning the transplant is not possible. A negative crossmatch means the antigens are compatible and a transplant is possible.

BLOOD TYPE COMPATABILITY			
DONORS		RECIPIENTS	
Blood Type	Donates to Type	Blood Type	Receives from Type
A	A, AB	A	A, O
B	B, AB	B	B, O
AB	AB	AB	A, B, AB, O
O	A, B, AB, O	O	O

RATE OF BLOOD TYPE FREQUENCY			
Blood Type	Rate of Frequency	Blood Type	Rate of Frequency
O	44%	B	10%
A	42%	AB	4%

Do I have to know someone who needs a kidney to donate?

The decision to donate a kidney is deeply personal and can be motivated in many ways. For some, it is a matter of helping a loved one whose kidneys are failing. Others may hear about someone more distant in dire need, like a co-worker or relative of a friend, and feel compelled to take action. And then there are those who are excited by the stories of everyday heroes who have donated to strangers and are inspired to do the same. Depending on the relation to their recipient, donors can be divided into two types: directed and nondirected.

Directed Donor

A directed donor gives their kidney to a specific recipient of their choice. Most donors today are directed.

Nondirected Donor

A nondirected donor is someone who donates without a chosen recipient. Other terms sometimes used to describe this type include *altruistic, anonymous, good Samaritan,* and *unspecified*. Nondirected donations make up only about 3% of all donations and are given to individuals on the national organ waitlist. Neither the donor nor the recipient receives information about the other. However, if both parties agree, some transplant centers may arrange for contact. Ask your transplant center in advance if this is an option if attempting recipient contact is important to you.

> Donations to strangers are rare. At the time of my donation, only three percent were non-direct (stranger) donations. What makes that three percent of donors so unique? Turns

out, there's a physiological reason. The amygdala is important for producing empathetic responses. Researcher Abigail Marsh found that altruistic donors had increased gray matter in that area. Apparently, my enlarged amygdala hardwired me."

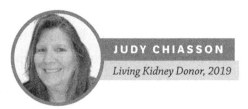

JUDY CHIASSON
Living Kidney Donor, 2019

What if I do not match my recipient?

Since around one-third of donors are not compatible with their recipients of choice,[91] exchange programs have been developed to make more transplants possible. Previously, people with kidney failure who did not have a compatible living donor had to wait for a deceased donor kidney, which could take years. The introduction of exchange programs has allowed living donors who are not compatible with their intended recipients to donate their kidneys to more compatible recipients, allowing their intended recipients to receive compatible kidneys. These exchange programs have been instrumental in helping more people get transplants and in a shorter amount of time.

Paired Exchange

In a paired exchange, each donor gives their kidney to another recipient who is a better match in exchange for a matched kidney for their intended recipi-

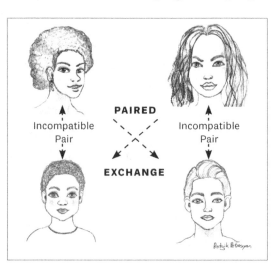

ent. Exchanges can repeat with multiple pairs. The surgeries may take place at the same hospital or different hospitals.

Chain Transplantation

Chain transplantation starts with a nondirected donor whose kidney goes to a recipient who has an incompatible donor, then that recipient's incompatible donor gives a kidney to another recipient with an incompatible donor. The chain continues until all recipients have received a compatible kidney. Chain transplantation is an exciting program that allows more people to receive transplants with better-matched kidneys.

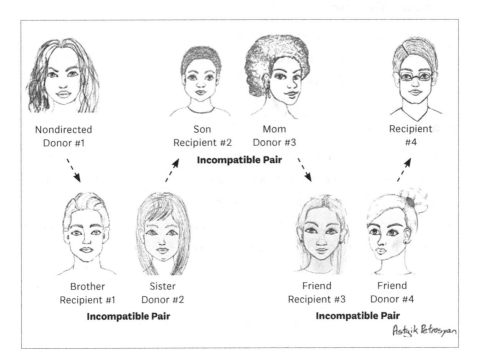

Can I donate now for a future transplant?

Advanced donation is another type of exchange where the donor receives a living donor kidney voucher in exchange for their donation. One recipient of their choice can use this voucher in the future if a kidney transplant is needed. It allows donors to donate before they are too old and at a time that is convenient for them. It is also useful for those who want to donate without a specific recipient in mind while safeguarding the possibility of donating to someone close to them in the future.

Standard Voucher

A standard voucher lets someone donate their kidney to a specific recipient who needs a transplant within a year, but the donor wants to donate before that time.

Family Voucher

The family voucher is for people who want to donate without a specific recipient in mind but want to protect their family's potential need for a kidney in the future. In exchange for the kidney donation, the donor may name up to five family members, and one of them may receive a living donor kidney in the future if needed.

Swap Saver

A swap saver is used when a paired recipient can no longer participate in a scheduled exchange due to an illness or other circumstances, and the donor decides to proceed with the donation to allow the rest of the exchange to take place. The paired recipient receives priority for a transplant in a future exchange when they are ready to proceed.

Real-Time Swap Failure

A real-time swap failure is when a paired donor completes a donation in an exchange program, but the intended recipient does not get a kidney transplant due to unforeseen circumstances. When this occurs, the intended recipient is prioritized for a future transplant in another exchange.[92]

If interested in participating in an exchange program, the following are ways to get started:

- Talk with your intended recipient's transplant center. Ask if an exchange program is a good option in your case.
- If a transplant center does not offer exchange programs, recipients may choose another transplant center that does.
- Contact these organizations that help facilitate exchanges: National Kidney Registry, OPTN/UNOS Kidney Paired Donation Program, and Alliance for Paired Donation.

> Before my daughter was diagnosed with kidney disease, I remember briefly considering kidney donation but was concerned that my parents or siblings would need my kidney in the future. Now with the voucher program, a main barrier to kidney donation for many people is eliminated. For our family, the voucher program came along at the perfect time. I was watching the progression of my daughter's kidney disease knowing that I may be considered too old to donate my kidney to her when she reached end stage kidney disease. The voucher program allowed me to donate my kidney to a recipient on the waiting list so that my daughter could have a voucher for a kidney from a living donor in the future when she needs it."

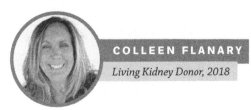

COLLEEN FLANARY
Living Kidney Donor, 2018

Can I Sell a Kidney?

The buying or selling of human organs for transplantation is a serious crime in nearly all countries and can have dangerous consequences for both the seller and the recipient. In addition to being illegal, selling organs often involves exploiting vulnerable individuals, such as those living in poverty, who may be coerced into selling their organs for financial gain and subjected to unsafe conditions. In the United States, buying or selling human organs for transplantation is a federal crime. This does not include the reimbursement for expenses, such as travel, housing, and lost wages incurred by the donor in connection with the donation.[93]

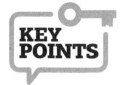

- Compatibility testing is essential to help prevent rejection.
- Donors may donate to a specific recipient, called directed donation, or to someone they do not know on the national kidney waitlist, called nondirected donation.
- Exchange programs make it possible for people with kidney failure to get transplants by swapping their incompatible donor with a compatible donor from another recipient.
- Voucher programs make it possible to donate in advance of a recipient's future transplant.

CHAPTER SIX

What Are the Health Risks of Donation?

Donating a kidney is a unique decision that will stay with you for the rest of your life, not one to take lightly. Before making this personal and significant choice, it is important to be aware and accept the potential risks involved with the surgery and any long-term impacts it can have on your health.

Fortunately, the risks for approved living kidney donors in the appropriate setting are considered low.[94] It is remarkable that kidney donors may continue to live a full and healthy life with little health impact. For many, donation even has a positive influence on their overall quality of life.[95,96,97]

However, it is important to recognize that while kidney donation is considered low-risk, it is not entirely risk-free. In addition to known risks, there are still some unknowns—*not all risks are thoroughly researched and understood.*

As you explore the possibility of becoming a donor, you may feel nervous when factoring the health risks into your decision. It's understandable to have concerns about how your gift may impact you, and appropriate to consider your willingness to accept them. When learning about health risks, you may feel more confident in your decision, or it may leave you feeling more hesitant. Either way, remember that to be approved to donate, you will undergo an extensive health evaluation where your transplant team looks for factors that may increase your chance of experiencing problems. If significant risk factors are found, you may be denied donation. This is for your protection. Your transplant team specializes in transplants and knows what to look for. They do not want complications any more than you do. If approved to donate, you can rest assured that your transplant team considers you safe to donate and that your risks are minimized.

 I felt the benefit far outweighed the risks. I looked at the success rates and said yes. It really was as simple as that."

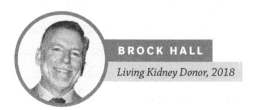

BROCK HALL
Living Kidney Donor, 2018

What are the immediate risks and potential complications?

Living donation is a major decision and involves certain health risks. As such, donors are required to sign an informed consent document that outlines the known complications that are possible. While the list is extensive and can feel daunting, it's important to note that the likelihood of these risks occurring is very low.

As when facing any major surgery, it is normal to be concerned. Surgery is never risk-free, even with every precaution taken. However, you may take some comfort in learning that the risks of kidney donation resulting in death is extremely rare, occurring at a rate of 0.03%, or 1 in 3,000.[98,99,100] While about 10% to 20% of donors receive a diagnosis or procedure for what is considered a minor complication of surgery,[101,102] these may just require a slightly longer hospital stay

WHAT ARE THE HEALTH RISKS OF DONATION? 61

or result in lingering symptoms after being discharged from the hospital. In rare cases, a major complication may require additional surgery or hospitalization to resolve, but major problems from surgery are reported to occur in only 3% to 5% of cases.[103,104,105]

> " The risks made me nervous, but my husband's health risks outweighed them. He was doing so poorly by then that it was affecting our whole family. He couldn't do daily activities without breaks and naps. I was willing to take the risk to have him back."

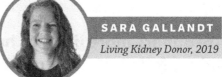

SARA GALLANDT
Living Kidney Donor, 2019

The surgery to remove a donated kidney is performed under general anesthesia, which puts you in a temporary deep sleep during the procedure. General anesthesia is considered safe and routinely used for surgeries worldwide. However, there is a small chance that the anesthesia procedure could cause problems ranging from mild and unpleasant to serious. Your healthcare team will take precautions to minimize the risk of any serious effects.

Most donors do not experience significant problems and only need to manage discomforts or infections. Stubborn constipation may cause cramping or sharp pain, and gas used to inflate the abdomen during most donor surgeries typically causes notable back or shoulder pain. Abdominal pain is common, but the intensity varies from donor to donor. Some describe it as mild and others more severe. In most cases, the pain subsides as the wounds heal. Chronic pain after the wound healing stage is possible, but not typical.[106]

Donating is a one-of-a-kind experience that can affect people in different ways. While some donors return to normal within days to weeks, others may require weeks to months to recover fully. In addition, it is quite common to feel exhausted, making it difficult to perform regular activities at home or work for an extended period. However, this fatigue typically fades as the body recovers.

Remember, your donor team wants you to have the best possible surgical experience and outcome, just like you do. Speak up if you experience any unexpected symptoms or have any concerns. Mild symptoms can sometimes indicate a bigger problem that needs medical attention. It is always better to address issues early.

Are donors more likely to have kidney failure in the future?

The development of kidney disease leading to kidney failure after donation is possible,[107] but the risk is considered very low. This is largely a result of the extensive donor evaluation. The rate of long-term kidney failure for donors at 15 years after donation is 0.31%, or about 1 in 300 compared to a failure rate of 0.04%, or about 1 in 2,500, in similarly healthy individuals.[108,109]

Young donors should consider additional age-related risk factors before deciding to donate. When evaluated as a kidney donor at a younger age, it is harder to predict the likelihood of developing kidney disease in the future. Kidney disease usually does not occur until middle age, and kidney failure is more common after age 60. It is also uncertain if a young donor will face other health issues that may be more difficult to treat with only one kidney.

Although kidney failure can occasionally occur after donation, it is not always related directly to the donation. The increased risk is primarily due to the development of other risk factors such as being overweight, high blood pressure, diabetes, or other unforeseen issues. Inherited diseases that were not detected during the medical evaluation may also contribute to future kidney failure in donors. However, using genetic testing as part of the health evaluation can reduce this risk.

> " I didn't focus on the risks which seemed minimal. I let the doctors decide what was safe and right for me and followed their lead."
>
> **ANDY GREENE**
> *Living Kidney Donor, 2017*

To assess the risk of future kidney failure, the eGFR value after donation is the best indicator in living kidney donors and can provide a clearer picture of any concerns.[110]

In the highly unlikely event kidney failure in the future occurs and a transplant is needed, donors are placed on the deceased kidney donor waitlist in a position that accounts for priority points given to living donors.[111]

How does living with one kidney affect me?

When living with just one kidney, the main difference is that you have less kidney function. While it may seem like you will be left with only half your pre-donation level, the good news is that the remaining kidney should increase in filtering capacity by way of hyperfiltration to compensate for some of the loss.[112]

Once the remaining kidney expands its function, most donors have about 25% to 35% less kidney function than pre-donation levels, although this may continue to improve slightly up to another 10% over three or so years.[113,114]

What does this reduced kidney function mean for you? Donors often end up with a level of kidney function after donation equivalent to mild to moderate kidney disease. However, if this is your experience, remember that you will not have kidney disease—you will have one healthy kidney! If you have been approved to donate, your donor healthcare team believes that your remaining kidney function will be sufficient for all that kidneys do for you.

However, it is impossible to predict what your experience will be. There are times when the remaining kidney does not compensate for the loss. And sometimes donors develop problems or experience limitations related to their donation. Examples of problems or limitations include the following.

Blood Pressure: Blood pressure may increase over time as a result of the changes that occurs in the remaining kidney after a donation.[115,116] Donors should have their blood pressure checked at least once yearly, and more frequently if rising blood pressure is detected.

Scarring: All surgeries carry some risks from scarring, both internally and externally. However, with the use of minimally invasive surgical techniques the risks are minimized. In rare cases, internal scars may form tough bands between abdominal tissues and organs that cause twisting and pulling sensations, obstructions, or pain. External scars may affect self-esteem and cause negative emotions like feeling less attractive or insecure. About 13% of donors have body image concerns due to scarring.[117]

Hernia: An incisional hernia is when tissue or organs push through the abdominal wall at the site of a surgical incision. Hernias can form after abdominal surgery, especially when too much physical activity, weight, or other increased pressure resumes before the surgical cuts are fully healed. Most hernias develop within three to six months but can develop at any time.[118,119] Hernias require surgery to repair.

Bone Disease: Bone health may be affected if parathyroid hormone changes after donation, decreasing essential minerals necessary for strong bones.[120,121,122,123] To prevent this, your healthcare provider may recommend routine blood tests, diet modification, moderate exercise, or nutritional supplementation if needed.

Fatigue: Sometimes donors experience lower energy levels that last 1 to 6 months.[124] The cause, prevalence, and duration are not yet clearly understood. While it is rare, some donors report having less energy years later.

Pregnancy: Kidney donors usually have normal pregnancies after donation, but there is a slightly increased risk for both the mother and the baby due to higher risks for preeclampsia and elevated blood pressure.[125,126] Discussing your desire for pregnancy with your transplant team is important. Pregnancy is not recommended for at least six months to one year after donation.[127] If you become pregnant, have a thorough prenatal care plan and monitor your blood pressure regularly.[128] Worth noting, some women have reported hormone-related changes after donation, though there are currently no studies to confirm the relation to donation. Work with your doctor if you experience concerning symptoms.

Gout: Gout is a type of painful arthritis caused by the buildup of uric acid in the joints. Living kidney donors may face an increased risk of gout due to decreased clearance of uric acid from the body.[129] Routine blood tests for elevated uric acid levels, known as hyperuricemia, may help in early detection and treatment to minimize potential complications.

Medication Limitations: Use of certain medications is limited when living with less kidney function. For example, nonsteroidal anti-inflammatory drugs (NSAIDs) used to reduce pain and inflammation are known to reduce blood flow to the kidneys and cause them harm if used regularly and are not recommended for kidney donors. In addition, a number of conditions may be harder to treat with less kidney function due to the toxicity of specific medications.[130]

> " I donated in 2014. My energy never returned, and I later developed an autoimmune disease that causes chronic pain, which I cannot treat with NSAIDs to get relief due to my kidney function level. There are many things to ponder and accept 100% before saying yes."

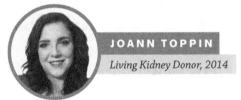

JOANN TOPPIN
Living Kidney Donor, 2014

Will my life be shorter if I donate?

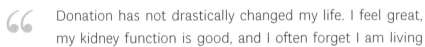

Living with one kidney or two does not appear to change life expectancy.[131] You can live the same number of years whether you donate or not.

> " Donation has not drastically changed my life. I feel great, my kidney function is good, and I often forget I am living with one kidney. That being said, I do have a greater respect for our bodies and their amazing capability to adapt."

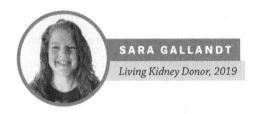

SARA GALLANDT
Living Kidney Donor, 2019

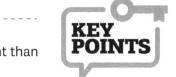

- Kidney donors typically feel no different than when they had two kidneys.
- Kidney donation is considered low-risk but is not risk-free, and not all health risks of living donation are known.
- Living donors can expect a normal life expectancy.
- In the rare event that a kidney donor needs a kidney transplant in the future, donors are assigned priority points on the kidney transplant waitlist for a deceased donor.

CHAPTER SEVEN

What Might I Expect From Surgery and Recovery?

Donating an organ can be an exciting experience. The opportunity to renew someone's health in such a profound way is amazing. Even so, as the big day approaches, nervousness and apprehension is completely normal and felt by most. Understanding what you might expect from the surgery and recovery may help you feel more prepared and keep you more at ease. When learning about the experiences of others and what you might expect, keep in mind, however, that every donation experience is unique. While some people bounce back quickly, others require more time. Since you cannot predict your experience, it is important to have a family or friend support system in place ready to help you for as long as you need it. With their assistance, you can take it easy and avoid complications that may arise from doing too much too soon. Having someone to talk to during your recovery can also provide emotional support and reassurance if your recovery is not what you anticipate or if you experience post-donation blues. Ultimately, being prepared helps to ensure a successful outcome and positive experience.

How should I prepare for the surgery?

You will receive specific instructions from your donor team about what to do and what not to do in preparation for surgery. It is crucial to follow these instructions carefully to help minimize risks. Following are some general guidelines of what you may expect:

- Stop smoking: Smoking increases the risk of cardiovascular and lung complications during surgery.
- Avoid alcohol.
- Do not take aspirin or pain relievers for seven days before surgery. These medications can increase the risk of bleeding.
- Do not take supplements like herbs and vitamins.

Blood transfusions during donor nephrectomies are very rare. However, if you wish to have your blood stored in case a transfusion is needed, talk to your healthcare team to make the arrangement.

Your donor team may ask you to provide advanced directives before the surgery. These forms are standard for any surgery. Advanced directives are legal documents that indicate your wishes for medical decisions in case you cannot make them yourself. You can find advanced directive forms online or get them from your transplant center.

How is it decided which kidney is donated?

Many factors are considered by the donor healthcare team when deciding which kidney to remove. These may include the size and function of the kidneys, the location of the kidneys in the body, and any irregularities of the kidneys. In most cases, the surgeon will choose the kidney that is easiest to access and leaves the donor with the more desirable kidney function. The decision is made on a case-by-case basis, with the health and well-being of the donor being the priority.

How is my kidney removed?

The surgical procedure to remove a healthy kidney from a living donor for transplantation into someone whose kidneys have failed is called a *donor nephrectomy*. There are essentially two methods for performing this surgery, laparoscopic and open. Both are equally successful. Your surgeon will discuss which method will be used before the surgery.

Laparoscopic Surgery

The laparoscopic method is the less invasive surgical technique. It requires less recovery time and is less painful than traditional open surgery.[132] Most donor nephrectomies today are performed laparoscopically. Laparoscopic surgery techniques vary among transplant centers and surgeons, but generally the surgeon makes a few small incisions in the abdomen and uses special tools and a camera to remove the kidney through a larger incision or a single-port method using one incision in the belly.[133] The laparoscopic method takes about 3 to 4 hours.

Open Surgery

The open method was the standard technique from the start of living kidney donation until the development of the laparoscopic approach. This method may be used if the laparoscopic method is not suitable for the donor or if problems arise during laparoscopic surgery. Open surgery is generally quicker than laparoscopic surgery, taking about 2 to 3 hours, but the recovery time is longer and more painful. Generally, the surgeon makes a 6 to 12-inch incision on one side of the abdomen, extending around the side of the body, where the kidney is removed.[134]

> " I was a little nervous going into surgery. I didn't know how my body was going to respond, what recovery would be like, how much pain there would be, etc. However, every time I started to feel those nerves, I thought of the person I was donating for having to spend their life battling kidney failure. I thought of the physical sickness and how frustrating that would have to be to fight day after day. I thought of them sitting for hours connected to dialysis and still not feeling good for long. Knowing that my sacrifice could stop that kind of suffering for years, maybe decades, was motivation enough for me to put my fears and anxiety aside. "

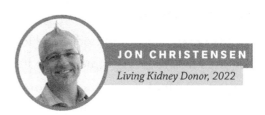

JON CHRISTENSEN
Living Kidney Donor, 2022

What is anesthesia?

Use of anesthesia is necessary for the surgery, which is a medical treatment that prevents pain and movement. It is administered by a specialized doctor called an anesthesiologist and consists of a combination of medication and inhaled gases which cause a state that feels like sleeping. After the surgery, the medication is reversed and the patient slowly wakes up in a recovery room. Some common side effects of anesthesia include grogginess, confusion, nausea, sore throat, shivering, or sleepiness, but these usually only last a few hours or maybe a day.

What happens after removing the kidney?

After removed from the donor, the kidney is prepared for transplantation or transportation. If the recipient is in the same hospital, the recipient's surgery will coincide with the donor's surgery and the kidney is placed into the recipient right away. If the recipient is at a different hospital, the kidney is prepared for immediate transportation.

Once the kidney is transplanted, it usually starts working soon after, but it may take a few days or weeks to function properly.

The hospital recovery time for a recipient is longer than for donors, usually around 5-7 days. The longer recovery is partly due to the risk of rejection, which is highest immediately after surgery. Signs of rejection are not uncommon, but this can usually be treated and resolved quickly.

If you are concerned about your recipient's progress after the transplant, talk openly with your healthcare team and ask questions to avoid undue stress that may impact your recovery experience.

How long will I be in the hospital?

The time spent in the hospital depends on the surgical method used and how quickly you recover. Most donors are released within 1 to 3 days, but the recovery period may be extended in some cases. There are several reasons why a donor may need more time to recover in the hospital than other donors, including:

- The use of open surgery instead of laparoscopic surgery
- Surgical complications
- Pain that is not well managed
- Difficulty urinating

Take your time and do not rush to leave the hospital. Allow the anesthesia to wear off and make sure any pain is manageable. Your donor team will also check to ensure that your remaining kidney is functioning well and monitor you for signs of internal bleeding or other issues. You will be released once your pain is under control, you can urinate normally, and there are no other signs of issues.

What do the scars look like?

The size and location of the scars depend on the surgical method and techniques used by the surgeon. Before the surgery, you will likely meet with your surgeon, where you may discuss the expected location and size of the scars. The extraction scar from where the kidney was removed will always be visible, but it will fade over time. Small scars where the camera and tools are inserted for laparoscopic surgeries typically become undetectable. It is not possible to know exactly what your scars will look like until you speak with your surgeon, but the following are examples of scars you might expect.

Laparoscopic Surgery

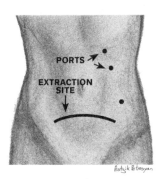

Laparoscopic surgery usually results in 2 to 3 small scars on the upper abdomen where the camera and tools are inserted and a scar about 3 to 4 inches long from the extraction site where the kidney was removed. Surgeons often try to place this incision low enough to be covered by clothing.

Hand-Assisted Laparoscopic Surgery

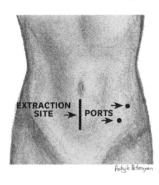

The hand-assisted laparoscopic method involves making an incision usually near the belly button through which the surgeon inserts a hand to remove the kidney. This method may also involve additional small incisions on the abdomen to insert the tools and camera.

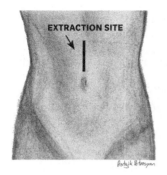

Single Site Laparoscopic Surgery

The single incision method leaves one scar near or encircling the belly button, similar to the hand-assisted laparoscopic scar, but it may be longer.

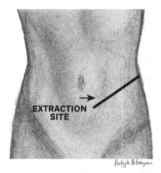

Open Surgery

Open surgery requires a longer incision placed higher on one side of the abdomen, typically measuring about 6 to 12 inches. This scar may take longer to heal and may be more visible long-term than the scars from laparoscopic methods.

What do I bring to the hospital?

Recovery time in the hospital is minimal, so there is no need to pack heavily. Plan to bring loose-fitting clothing that will not irritate the incision to wear when leaving the hospital. You may also want to bring a robe or sweater, slip-on shoes or slippers for walking around the hospital halls, and a warm blanket and socks to stay comfortable if the hospital room is chilly. A small bag of toiletries, such as lotion, a hairbrush, toothbrush, toothpaste, baby wipes, and lip balm may be useful to freshen up. If you usually wear contacts, bring your glasses. Remember to pack any medications you regularly take and bring enough to last a few days longer than your planned hospital stay in case your recovery takes a little longer than expected. You may also want to bring a phone and extra-long charging cord, earphones for music or videos to help pass the time, and earplugs to help you relax or sleep while recovering. A small, firm pillow or abdomen binder can be helpful to support the abdomen and lessen the pain when you move, cough, sneeze, laugh, or wear a seatbelt when leaving the hospital. Finally, leaving any valuable items at home or with someone accompanying you at the hospital is best.

Do I need a caregiver?

Plan to have a caregiver for at least the first few days after surgery, preferably the first two weeks, to help with everyday tasks and ensure your safety. This may include getting your medications, helping to change clothes, and shifting positions in bed. A caregiver may also provide meals, run errands, and lift anything heavier than post-surgical weight restrictions. Help is especially essential for those with children or animals who need care. After two weeks, you should be able to take care of your daily needs but may still need assistance with young children and lifting anything over recovery weight restrictions.

> Give yourself time to heal. Listen to the advice your medical team gives you. Do what they say even when you don't want to. Gather a team of friends and family to support you when you come home. We had meals set up for a couple of weeks, and friends doing yard work. It was a life saver."

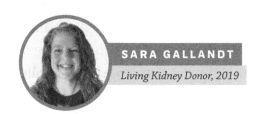

SARA GALLANDT
Living Kidney Donor, 2019

What are signs that I should contact the transplant center?

If you notice any concerning changes, even if they seem minor, contact your transplant center. Getting early treatment for a developing issue can help prevent significant problems. You should receive a list of symptoms to watch for when discharged from the hospital. Generally, symptoms that are a sign that you need medical help include:

- Fever
- Shortness of breath or difficulty breathing
- Leg swelling
- Worsening pain
- A red streak near the incision
- Drainage from the incision
- Cloudy or strong-smelling urine
- Urinating more frequently
- Burning during urination
- Vomiting

Will I need to return to the transplant center for checkups?

Follow-up care varies depending on the transplant center. Some centers ask donors to return for a checkup in a week or two. When donors live far, they may be required to stay nearby for a few days to two weeks to test and monitor their health. Others might arrange for testing close to home or telehealth visits.

Some donors report feeling disconnected from the transplant center after completing their donation. This is normal because the donation is over and the need to be seen by the transplant center is less. However, transplant centers are concerned about the long-term health of their donors. Donors should always reach out to their center if they think there is something wrong that is related to the donation or have questions. If you do not get a sufficient response, *do not ignore the need for monitoring or concerning symptoms. Instead, seek care elsewhere, if needed.*

How will I feel during the recovery?

After surgery, you can expect at least some degree of discomfort. The amount of discomfort experienced is unpredictable and varies from person to person. Some donors experience very little discomfort while others experience significant pain. Common types of discomfort described by donors during their recovery include pain, gas and bloating, constipation, nausea, tiredness, and discomfort around the incision.

> My recovery initially was very difficult. I was warned that it would be, but it still surprised me. My kidney did not work right away in my husband. That hit me hard and affected my recovery. It kicked in a day or so later, but it was a difficult time. Once I got over the first few days, movement was key. The more I moved the better I felt."

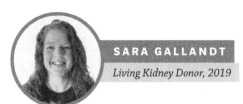

SARA GALLANDT
Living Kidney Donor, 2019

LEARN MORE

Navigating Common Recovery Discomforts

Pain

It is natural to feel pain after a major surgery like removing a kidney. However, the intensity and duration can vary significantly. Common types of pain donors experience include:

- Bloating and gas
- Painful constipation
- Sharp or stabbing pain in the abdomen or shoulders
- Testicular swelling
- Nerve pain that may run down the thigh

Your healthcare team will help manage your pain and may prescribe medications for use at home. In addition, some donors find the following techniques helpful for easing discomfort during recovery:

- Walking
- Visits from family or friends to distract you
- Heating pad
- Ice pack
- Small pillow or abdominal binder to compress the abdomen
- Music or movies to keep you distracted
- Gentle stretching
- Light massage
- Games
- Meditation or prayer

Gas and Bloating

After laparoscopic surgery, gas and bloating are typical for about a week. This is caused by the carbon dioxide used during surgery to inflate the abdomen.

The body eventually absorbs and releases this gas, but until it does, it can cause pressure and discomfort in the gut. You may also experience sharp shoulder pain due to the gas hitting a nerve that runs from the abdomen to the neck. Walking is often helpful to encourage the gas to be absorbed more quickly and reduce discomfort.

Constipation

Constipation is one of the most common complaints after surgery. It can be caused by anesthesia, manipulation of the bowels during surgery, and pain medications that can slow down bowel movements. This can make it difficult to pass stool and may lead to pain if gas and stool become trapped. You may be prescribed stool softeners while in the hospital. However, before starting any over-the-counter stool softeners or laxatives, be sure to consult with your healthcare team. If constipation persists, it may take some time and a combination of remedies to regain regular bowel movements. Following are suggestions donors find helpful:

- Walk as much as you are safely able each day.
- Drink a lot of fluids to keep stool soft.
- Drink warm prune juice (boil prunes in water, drink the liquid, and eat the prunes).
- Drink hot peppermint tea.
- Eat high-fiber foods, such as apples, berries, raw veggies, and oats.

Nausea

Nausea is common after surgery. It is typically caused by anesthesia and pain medications. If you experience this, medications may be offered to help calm it down. You may also find minimizing the use of pain medication helpful to reduce or prevent nausea.

Tiredness

It is normal to feel fatigued due to surgical trauma and the immediate loss of half your kidney function. The tiredness can range from mild

WHAT MIGHT I EXPECT FROM SURGERY AND RECOVERY?

to severe. Mild drowsiness may not greatly impact your days, while exhaustion may require you to sleep more or adjust how much you do daily. It is important to give your body the rest it needs. Gentle exercise can help, but it is essential to avoid overdoing it. Fatigue may last for weeks or months and, in rare cases, longer.

Incision Discomfort
Discomfort or strange sensations around the incision area or down the thigh is common. These symptoms are caused by the cutting of nerves during the surgery and will gradually improve as the nerves regenerate. These sensations may include burning, numbness, tingling, itching, or other unusual feelings.

> Post-surgery, my mantra was "Something new every day." From the time I woke up from surgery, I always made an effort to do something new. Those first days "something new" may have been simply putting on my socks by myself or walking an extra lap in the hospital. But every day I saw myself doing something new I also saw myself getting better and stronger. Seeing that progress was important, mentally, for me. And it's become a new standard in my life now that I feel totally recovered. "

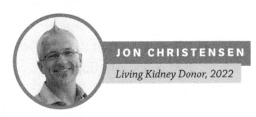

JON CHRISTENSEN
Living Kidney Donor, 2022

How long does it take to get back to normal activities?

The first two weeks will be the most challenging part of your recovery. It is also when you need to be the most cautious and restricted. During this time, it is important to rest and take it easy. Engage in low-energy activities, such as reading, listening to music, or watching movies. Gradually increase your activity levels as your body allows. Most donors find that their discomfort begins to resolve within 1 to 3 weeks and that they can mostly return to their regular routines within in 4 to 6 weeks with some adjustments.

It was very painful for a couple of days, but I quickly recovered and was back to normal in about 6 weeks."

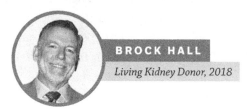

BROCK HALL
Living Kidney Donor, 2018

However, some donors take longer to recover, especially if they experience post-surgical complications that require an extended hospital stay, readmission to the hospital, or a surgical procedure. Even after returning to regular activities, some donors continue to experience fatigue, weakness, discomfort, or mood fluctuations for several months to a year, or longer in rare cases.

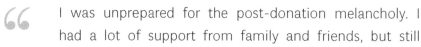

I was unprepared for the post-donation melancholy. I had a lot of support from family and friends, but still had low mood. It lasted about two-weeks and improved in sync with my physical recovery."

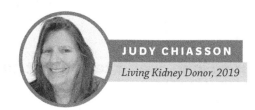

JUDY CHIASSON
Living Kidney Donor, 2019

Since the recovery time can vary from person to person, it is important to have a plan in place in case you need more time to fully recover than expected. This helps to avoid overdoing it and causing a problem. Preparing for your recovery can help ensure that it goes smoothly and successfully.

Talk to your healthcare team about your recovery expectations and let them know if your recovery is taking longer than expected. Additionally, ask about safe ways to return to activities that are important to you. As your healing progresses, you should be able to do more each day.

Lifting Heavy Objects

Weight restrictions are a critical part of a successful recovery. Your incision will heal on the surface quickly, but the deeper tissues take significantly longer. Lifting heavy objects before these tissues have time to heal can result in a hernia, a protrusion of tissue through the inner abdominal wall near the incision site. Hernias require surgery to repair and can be painful. A common sign that you have a hernia is a bulge near the surgery scar. They usually develop within the first couple months after surgery but can develop after years.

To avoid problems caused by weight, avoid lifting anything over 10 to 15 pounds for about 4 to 6 weeks or as instructed by your healthcare team. That is roughly the same weight as a medium cat or a laundry basket of towels. After that, avoid heavy lifting, pulling, and twisting for about eight weeks. This may include activities like carrying children, doing chores like heavy gardening, walking your dog, and lifting weights at a gym. Even if your feel back to normal, it is crucial to allow your body plenty of time to heal before returning to strenuous activities to avoid issues.

Work

The amount of time it takes to return to work varies depending on your type of job and rate of recovery. For instance, jobs involving physical labor, such as construction or horse training, can take longer than mental jobs, like coding or accounting. Generally, people are back on the job within 2 to 6 weeks, but it can take longer if the work is physically demanding or the healing process is slower than expected.

> Listen to your body and take as much time as you need to recover. Don't overdo it when you start to feel better. Let people help as much as they're willing. I took 4 weeks off work, but 5 or 6 could have been better. It takes time to get your stamina back."

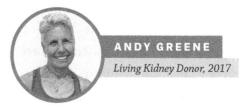

ANDY GREENE
Living Kidney Donor, 2017

Driving

Driving is best avoided for at least a week or two, and sometimes longer, due to the use of anesthesia, pain medications, as well as the movements required to operate a vehicle. Steering, shifting, accelerating, and braking can put pressure on the incision and cause problems. Additionally, driving too soon may be a safety hazard since you may not have the abdominal strength to lift your leg and stop quickly.

Swimming and Bathing

Swimming and soaking in a tub or spa should be avoided until the incision has completely healed, generally about three weeks.

Exercise and Sports

Exercising can be beneficial for your recovery. Walking is an effective way to help your bowels move and promote blood circulation, both of which can improve the healing process. However, take it slow and gradually increase the distance as your body allows. It is critical to refrain from strenuous exercise until you fully recover to prevent problems. Your donor team can inform you when you are ready to participate in normal activities, usually within 4 to 8 weeks or so.

Diet

While there are no specific dietary restrictions directly related to kidney donation, it is still important to eat a healthy diet to maintain good health and avoid any future kidney-related problems. Avoid drinking alcohol until advised it is safe to do so. Additionally, it is crucial to stay well hydrated by drinking *at least* the recommended daily requirements of water for your body size. See Chapter 10 for more about hydration and eating healthy when living with one kidney.

Sexual Activity

Sexual activity that is not too physically demanding may be resumed once you feel ready, but you should avoid activities that are especially physical for at least 4 to 6 weeks or longer while your abdomen is healing.

Pregnancy

Talk to your obstetrician and donor team before trying to get pregnant. It's usually recommended to wait at least six months, and preferably one year, before attempting to have children for the safety of both the mother and baby.[135,136,137]

Take your recovery very seriously. It is as serious as the recipient's recovery. Recovery took longer than expected."

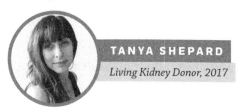

TANYA SHEPARD
Living Kidney Donor, 2017

How do I care for the incision?

You will receive specific instructions when leaving the hospital about how to take care of your incision at home. Generally, you will be instructed to keep it clean and dry, only using soap and water or products recommended by the hospital. Do not submerge in a bath or pool until the visible incisions are entirely healed.

What can I do for incision pain?

Discomfort around the area of the incision is normal and expected. To reduce pressure and pain, try holding a small, stiff pillow firmly against the incision area or loosely wearing an abdominal binder. For the first few days, you may want to use an ice pack up to 15 minutes at a time to reduce swelling and provide relief. Once the swelling has gone down, you may want to use a warm heating pad at short intervals to help with the remaining discomfort. Elevate your head and upper body while lying down to reduce pressure on the incision. Tell your donor team if the incision shows signs of infection, including pus or drainage, a bad smell, redness, hot to the touch, worsening pain, or if you develop a fever.

"The pain was intense, but I knew the whole time it was worth it, and it would go away. That made all the difference. My recipient and I spent the first week texting and trying not to laugh."

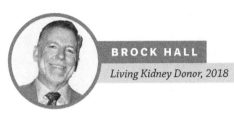

BROCK HALL
Living Kidney Donor, 2018

Will I need to take medications?

Donors do not take any long-term medications related to kidney donation. Pain medication during the first week or so is usually welcomed but not required. If you were to develop an infection, you would be prescribed antibiotics.

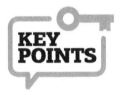

KEY POINTS

- The surgical and recovery experience can be very different between donors.
- Talk to your surgeon in advance about any questions, such as the scars you might expect or the surgery method used.
- It is important to give your body plenty of time to heal without rushing back to normal activities. Caregivers and advance planning can help you avoid doing too much too soon and causing unnecessary pain, setbacks, or issues.

CHAPTER EIGHT

Will Donating Cost Financially?

The life-giving gift of organ donation is a truly generous and valuable act. As such, the medical costs of organ donation are not the responsibility of the donor. In most countries, donors incur no financial responsibility. In the U.S., the recipient's healthcare insurance covers the medical and travel expenses for organ donation in most cases. However, there are times when donors may incur some financial loss,[138] such as when a recipient's insurance does not cover all medical or travel expenses or when financial hardship is experienced due to time off work, especially if the recovery takes longer than anticipated.

To help eliminate the financial impact and barrier to living organ donation, nearly half of the states in the U.S. allow tax deductions or credits for donor expenses.[139] In addition, generous charitable organizations offer financial reimbursement to donors who meet specific eligibility guidelines. Contact the organizations providing financial support listed in the Donor Resources section of this guidebook to find out what you may qualify to receive.

Learning about the potential costs of donating and what aid may be available can help you plan and avoid any financial strain from your charitable gift.

What will the evaluation team want to know about my finances?

Reviewing your financial stability is part of the donor evaluation to help assure that donating your kidney will not leave you with undue financial strain. You will be asked money-related questions to help the team determine if kidney donation may impact you financially. Questions you may be asked include:

- What is your line of work? Do you have a physically demanding job that will require more time off?
- Are you the sole provider for your family?
- Will your employer allow you to take a flexible number of weeks off?
- How will time off work impact your ability to pay bills?
- Do you have enough savings to cover lost wages and make your bill payments on time?
- Do you have health insurance?
- How will you pay for your future kidney checkups or any healthcare treatment, if needed?
- Who will assist you with your recovery? Do you need to pay for this assistance?
- Do you have children or animals who will need assistance? Do you need to pay for this assistance?

What medical costs are covered by my recipient's insurance?

All medical costs directly related to the donor evaluation and surgery are billed to and should be paid by your recipient's health insurance. Covered medical costs usually include the following:

- Donor evaluation medical tests
- Surgery
- Hospital stay for recovery
- Short-term follow-up care

What medical costs might be my responsibility?

It may not always be clear what expenses a donor may encounter. However, your transplant center can help you understand what medical expenses are covered and what may not be covered by your recipient's health insurance. It is a good idea to learn about these potential expenses in advance so that you can prepare accordingly, especially if you do not have health insurance. To get a better understanding of donor expenses and if any assistance is available for specific donor expenses, talk with your transplant center.

Expenses typically not covered by a recipient's health insurance include the following:

Preventative Screenings

Preventative screenings may be required during a donor evaluation. While these tests are often not covered by the recipient's insurance, they are usually covered by a donor's health insurance. Examples of preventative screenings that may be required during the donor evaluation include a colonoscopy, mammogram and pelvic exam for women, and a prostate exam for men.

Unrelated Medical Treatment

If medical issues are found during the evaluation, and you receive treatments unrelated to the donation for these issues, the costs for treatments are not paid for by the recipient's insurance.

Medical Complications

Medical problems after the surgery may or may not be covered by a recipient's insurance. It is sometimes unclear if any issues that occur after donation are directly related to the donation and left to interpretation by the transplant center or the recipient's insurance. Sometimes transplant centers will help with these expenses when appropriate.

What about any future medical expenses?

After discharged from the hospital, routine follow-up lab tests and medical visits (scheduled by the transplant center) are typically covered by the recipient's insurance for up to two years, though this is not always the case. It is important to note that all other costs become the donor's responsibility. If you have health insurance, it should cover future medical expenses. However, without health insurance, these expenses are up to you. Examples of future medical expenses include:

- Lifetime routine checkups
- Long-term medical care if the donation causes any problems

What if I do not have insurance?

Some transplant centers require donors to have health insurance before donating. However, even if yours does not, you may want to consider carrying health insurance in the unlikely event you experience medical problems. In addition, all future preventative kidney checkups and any other care after the donation are at your expense, but health insurance may make these medical expenses more affordable.

Will I be able to get insurance after donation?

Not long ago, donors often faced discrimination from insurance companies. Fortunately, there have been significant strides in recent years to protect living donors. In the U.S., the Affordable Care Act prevents health insurance companies from denying coverage or charging higher premiums to people with pre-existing conditions, including organ donation. While some types of insurance, like life insurance, long-term care insurance, and disability insurance, may still be more difficult or expensive to obtain for organ donors, ongoing efforts are addressing this issue. For example, the Living Donor Protection Act, currently pending in Congress, would prohibit discrimination against organ donors by insurance companies. Additionally, some states have already passed laws to protect organ donors from insurance discrimination. Check the status of your state to see if it has such protections in place.

> Do not take the financial aspects lightly. Take the assistance that is offered by donor assistance programs, friends, and family. There are costs that may creep up that are unexpected, but it is worth it."

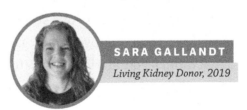

SARA GALLANDT
Living Kidney Donor, 2019

How much time off work will I need ?

When considering organ donation, it is important to plan for the potential financial impact of lost wages. The amount of time needed off work to recover from donation varies among donors. Some return to work in 2 to 6 weeks, while others need longer. Consider the physical demands of your job and the risks of returning to work too soon. If you have a strenuous job, you may need to take more time off work to avoid complications from abdominal surgery, which would require even more time off for recovering from the setback.

Talk to your employer about your donation plans and discuss a flexible timeframe for returning to work. Your employer may be able to offer support and accommodations to help you recover safely. Find out if your job is secure even if you need more time than is expected.

Do I have legal rights to time off work for donation?

The Family Medical Leave Act (FMLA) in the United States provides qualified workers with up to 12 weeks of unpaid, job-protected leave for living organ donation. Federal government employees are entitled to 30 days of paid leave for organ donation, as well as their standard sick and annual leave. Many states also offer state employees up to 30 days of paid or unpaid leave for living organ donation recovery, and some have extended leave policies for living organ donors in the private sector. Check with your state for current medical leave policies and talk to your employer about your specific leave options. The National Kidney Foundation has useful information about state medical leave policies on their website at kidney.org.

Can I get financial help from my employer?

You may be eligible for financial assistance to help cover the costs of time away from work during the surgery and recovery. Some states have programs that entitle employees to paid time off for living donation, while others offer tax credits. You can also check with your employer to see if your employee benefits package includes options like paid time off for organ donation, paid vacation, short-term disability, or sick leave that can help with your expenses while you are not receiving a paycheck.

> My employer was good to work with me, but I still needed to use my paid time off and didn't have enough to cover the surgery and recovery. Thankfully, my nurse coordinator told me about National Living Donor Assistance Center (NLDAC). I was hesitant initially because I didn't want to add costs to anyone for a decision I was making. However, after reading their website and asking some questions, I applied and received a generous assistance offer. The staff was great to work with there, and they moved very quickly so that I didn't have to worry about any finances as a result of my donation. I would absolutely suggest that every donor learn about what financial relief is available to them."

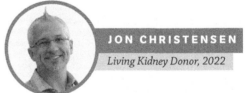

JON CHRISTENSEN
Living Kidney Donor, 2022

Can living donation affect future employment or career choices?

Living with one kidney may, though rarely, impact career choices—especially careers that are highly physical. For example, some branches of military service, police, and fire departments may not accept someone with one kidney.[140] If you have a physical career or desire to start one, check with the governing organization to be sure there are no disqualifying factors related to living with one kidney.

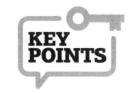

- Living organ donation is an exceptionally generous gift. However, donors may still incur financial expenses.

- Advance financial planning and arrangements with your employer may help minimize any financial impact on you or your family.

- Donor assistance programs help to eliminate any financial barriers to living donation.

CHAPTER NINE

What Emotions Might I Expect to Feel?

Donating a kidney can be an incredibly fulfilling and rewarding experience. Impacting a life in such a profound way often leaves donors feeling purposeful, proud, and grateful. It is not unusual for donors to declare that donating was one of the best things they have ever done. While the full psychosocial outcome is not entirely clear, 90% of donors are satisfied with life after donation.[141] Even when the recipient experiences an unfavorable outcome, 97% of donors report not regretting their decision to donate and would make the same decision to donate again.[142] Despite any challenges faced during or after donation, research has shown that most living kidney donors consider their experience as positive and their quality of life has either remained the same or improved.[143,144,145]

However, organ donation can also be an emotional journey, and donors may experience a range of unexpected feelings, especially if the outcome or experience of donation is not as anticipated. Even when the transplant is successful and donors recover as presumed, they may still feel drained and overwhelmed by the emotional highs and lows of the experience.

It is important to be aware of your emotions during the donation process and remember that they are normal and valid. Being emotionally aware simply means recognizing, respecting, and accepting your feelings as they come. This doesn't mean you have to dwell on your emotions. Rather, take a moment to pause, notice, and consider how to address them productively. Being emotionally aware and prepared may help you:

- Pause to think before reacting to difficult emotions.
- Notice and identify what triggers difficult emotions.
- Avoid or resolve conflicts in a healthy way.
- Get past complicated feelings more easily.
- Use healthy coping strategies to manage difficult emotions.
- Be less self-critical and more kind to yourself.

What are the emotional benefits of donating?

We all know the importance of giving and how it helps those in need. But it's not just recipients who benefit from volunteering, making financial contributions, or something as extraordinary as donating organs. Evidence shows that giving can satisfy fundamental human desires, including the need for purpose, community, self-esteem, and happiness.[146] In fact, many donors find the experience of giving the gift of life transformational, leading to improved overall well-being and optimism.[147,148,149] For some, the power to improve the lives of others is considered a privilege that enhances their self-esteem and personal growth.[150]

In addition to the personal advantages, giving can also bring people closer together. When we give to others, we often feel a deeper connection to them, and they feel closer to us. This can be especially true in the case of organ donation, where the donor, recipient, and their families and communities are all impacted by the act of giving.[151] As a result, the experience of organ donation can forge bonds and create a sense of unity and solidarity.

It is said that we increase our love by giving it away. When we love others, it often returns to us in greater measure.

> It is one of the most beautiful compensations of life that no man can sincerely try to help another without helping himself.
>
> RALPH WALDO EMERSON

> At the young age of 22 years (1977), I became a living kidney donor to my brother. At that time, and even now, that act does not stand out as a big deal. I probably wasn't even thinking about it much because when a family is in a crisis, there cannot be hesitation or second thoughts. We do what's needed. So, it was a spontaneous act. But the returns I got from that donation have been fantastic. My life has been immensely blessed. It has connected me with many wise and helpful people, and overall I have been living a comfortable and joyful family life.
>
> Fast forward to 2010: I went for my kidney function evaluation and was diagnosed with stage 3 chronic kidney disease. After that, my kidney function progressively went down, and by early 2016, I started peritoneal dialysis, a home treatment with a machine. For any organ transplant, finding a matching organ is a big deal. Living donors are hard to find, and to get a matching deceased organ anywhere in California, the queue is more than 10 years! So, I had to broaden my search. Within a short 3 months of registering with a small hospital in 2018 in Texas, I received my call for a transplant offer.

Every day I salute and pray for my unknown donor, who has reinforced my belief that *we are all connected as one human race with invisible bonds of love and compassion for each other."*

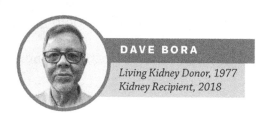

DAVE BORA
Living Kidney Donor, 1977
Kidney Recipient, 2018

How do I know if I am emotionally ready to donate?

Before making your decision to donate, take time to honestly assess where you are emotionally and what you can handle. Donating for the right reasons, at the right time, and with realistic expectations is important. Reflect on how donation might impact you during and after the process. If you are already grappling with issues like depression, anxiety, or a lack of support, these concerns could intensify after donation. If going through a divorce or other major life-stressors, the timing may not be right for you. If you are unsure about your emotional readiness, it can be helpful to confide in someone you trust, such as a family member, friend, religious or spiritual advisor, counselor, or someone who has donated before. Talking to people other than your intended recipient can help you sort through any worries and come to a decision.

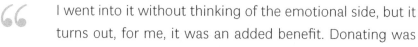

" I went into it without thinking of the emotional side, but it turns out, for me, it was an added benefit. Donating was the best thing I've done. It makes me feel like I got to do something extremely meaningful with my life, beyond what I expected."

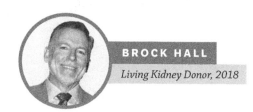

BROCK HALL
Living Kidney Donor, 2018

How might donating be hard emotionally?

Donating a kidney can be an intense and complex emotional experience, especially when someone close to you suffers from the pain and worry of kidney failure. It is natural to feel guilty for being healthy while a loved one is not or feel pressure to help. Reluctant donors who feel an obligation to donate may experience stress, worry, and even anger. Other times, donors may feel pressure from family members who are against the donation, especially to someone who is not a part of the family. This can be a difficult situation for the donor, who may feel torn between their desire to help the recipient and their desire to have the support of their family. For some donors, family members may be concerned about the risks of surgery and potential long-term effects of having only one kidney. Others may worry about a family member possibly needing the kidney donation themselves in the future, which may also create jealousy or resentment towards the recipient. Furthermore, the family may worry about a donor's health and well-being and may not understand why they would undergo elective surgery to donate a kidney to someone else.

These concerns can create uncertainty for the donor, causing them to question whether they are making the right decision. It can also create tension and conflict within the family and make the donor feel isolated and unsupported. This clash sometimes resolves when donors educate their family members about the donation process and the risks involved and invite them to attend donor evaluation appointments. Getting the family involved may help ease concerns and foster understanding and support.

Unfortunately, the recovery process can also create challenging emotions for donors as it is possible they may face a depressed mood. This can be caused by a variety of factors, such as the effects of anesthesia or the trauma of surgery, as well as discomfort, fatigue, or weakness that prevents them from engaging in the physical activities they enjoy. Difficult emotions may also arise if the experience does not meet their expectations. Donors with a history of depression are at a higher risk for depression after donation. Mood disturbance affects about 16% of donors.[152,153,154]

The emotional complexities of living organ donation can run deep and be compounded by a recipient's response to the gift. While donors do not give with the expectation of receiving in return, it can still feel hurtful and disappointing when the sacrifice goes unrecognized. It's like giving away a treasured possession to someone you hoped would cherish it, then it turns out they don't appear to value it as much as you do. Altruistic intentions can become overshadowed by a lack of demonstrated appreciation and dampen the giving experience.

Donating an organ to a stranger can lead to disappointment if the recipient doesn't want to know their donor or acknowledge the gift with gratitude. Lack of recognition can be especially painful if it comes from loved ones. When the receiver of the kidney is a spouse, the tangles of the relationship can provoke discomfort even further. Recipients may feel thankful for the gift of life but also may experience guilt and indebtedness to their donor. Coping with their illness, transplant, and related emotions like mortality and dependence can be overwhelming. This may lead to avoiding more tricky emotions, like acknowledging the suffering or hardships their donor may have endured to give them a new lease on life. Donor-recipient emotional relationships are complex and can be challenging to unravel.

> " I had a rollercoaster of emotions. Different communication styles can make this surgery very challenging. I was disappointed that my husband didn't express the appreciation the way I needed. I longed for something more affectionate. He doesn't show emotion so strongly, so his expression didn't feel

genuine. I partly gave out of love. The other part was out of sacrifice, and for that I felt the need for recognition. But maybe my primary reason was actually selfish—I didn't want to live without him!"

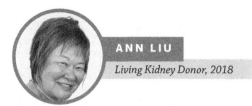

ANN LIU
Living Kidney Donor, 2018

The situation can become even more complicated when a donor and recipient live together. Recipients must typically take immunosuppressant medications to prevent organ rejection in higher doses immediately after the transplant, which can cause a range of side effects at this level, including mood swings and changes in behavior. At the same time, the donor might be dealing with challenges like pain and worry. When both experience mood changes after the surgery, this can amplify any existing conflicts and strain the relationship. Therefore, it is important to be aware of the potential for changes in both parties, communicate openly and honestly to manage relational challenges, and seek professional support to avoid ongoing conflict or lasting harm to the relationship.

Occasionally, donors experience regret, resentment, or life dissatisfaction. These emotions are more likely to occur if the donated organ does not function after being transplanted, if rejected early on, or if medical problems arise for the donor or recipient.[155] Similarly, if the recipient's life is not extended for as long as hoped or the relationship with the recipient declines, disappointment and remorse may emerge.[156,157] A significant 21% of donors experience fear of kidney failure for themselves.[158]

Remember that while it is natural to feel a range of emotions before, during, and after donation, seeking support can help you navigate complicated emotions and ultimately enhance your overall experience.

> I'm sure we all start the donation process because we want to improve someone's life. In my case, my recipient had been on dialysis for 10 years. She couldn't travel or enjoy so much of the life she used to know. She was getting weaker and her partner, my friend, was more and more in a caregiver role, so their relationship was affected.
>
> So, I had a picture of what a new kidney would mean to them and their future. After the surgery, she was doing great. She had 6 good months, feeling healthy and stronger, going back to work, and feeling optimistic about her future for the first time in many years. Then I got the news that she had cancer and was going to need surgery. They didn't want to tell me at first because they thought I would be sorry I donated. It hit me hard, and I was so sad for them that they had so little time before this happened. I was never sorry, but I had to let go of my story of how this was supposed to go. I found myself reassuring them that I was ok and that they should focus on her health.
>
> As it turned out, my recipient lived 5 more years, but she battled various forms of cancer for all those years. There was chemo, radiation, more surgery, etc., and all through it, they told me the kidney was good and it had made all the treatments possible.
>
> When the kidney was finally failing, I was the one comforting them when they thought I would be upset. My recipient felt she had let me down. So many times during her treatments, she said she stayed strong because she wanted the kidney to survive.

My recipient passed away in July of 2022. She never had to go back on dialysis, but her body was too tired to continue. I wish I could have done more to help her, and I was so sorry that the road had been so hard. She reassured me at the end that I had given her the extra 5 ½ years and she was never sorry she had the transplant.

When I attended her funeral, her friends and family thanked me for helping her. Only after the burial did I feel the loss of a part of me forever. Before that, the kidney belonged to someone else, and I didn't feel it was mine.

It's definitely a mixture of feelings that are unique to this situation and the relationship between a donor and recipient. It wasn't the happy ending I hoped for, but I know I made a difference for her and her family and friends, and I would do it again, without a doubt."

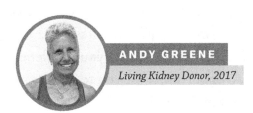

ANDY GREENE
Living Kidney Donor, 2017

" It was several months before my recipient responded to my annual kidney-versary email. She dreaded telling me that our kidney did not survive her chemotherapy. Of course, I was positive and supportive, but my ensuing cacophony of feelings confused me. My sadness exceeded my concern for my recipient. I had donated my kidney with the hope (but not guarantee) that it would bring a long life to my recipient. Besides, as an advance donor my primary recipient still had his valid voucher, so that was secure. Yet I felt such turmoil. I finally asked to meet with my organ coordinator who is a licensed social worker. She helped me sort out my feelings and see that my donation was not in vain. I came to feel grateful that my strong kidney sustained my recipient through her chemotherapy. Calling my donation coordinator was very wise. The specialists in the organ donation centers are uniquely knowledgeable with valuable resources to address the emotional aspects of kidney donation."

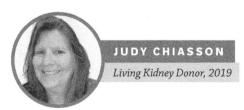

JUDY CHIASSON
Living Kidney Donor, 2019

What is the psychosocial evaluation?

During the psychosocial assessment portion of the donor evaluation, a psychiatrist, psychologist, or social worker with transplant experience will ask questions to determine if there are any emotional concerns that may cause you problems after your donation. This is also an opportunity for you to discuss any hesitations, fears, or pressures you may feel. Talking over your feelings ahead of time may help you avoid any emotional or relational problems in the future. Anything you discuss during this evaluation will remain confidential between you and your donor team. Examples of questions that may be asked during the psychosocial evaluation include the following.[159]

Pressure to Donate

Is someone pressuring you to donate? Are you being bribed with money, recognition, or anything of value? Will you feel guilty if you don't donate?

> Do not donate out of guilt. I cannot express this enough. The surgery is a risk, and no one should take that risk under guilt. My team was amazing and always told me that they would give me an out if I decided I didn't want to donate. If you are feeling under pressure, ask your donor team to give you an out without others knowing the reason. No one should donate unless they want to."

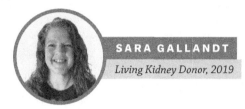

SARA GALLANDT
Living Kidney Donor, 2019

Pain Tolerance

How well do you tolerate pain? Do you have healthy ways to cope?

Support for Your Decision to Donate

Are your family and close friends supportive or against your decision to donate? Are they worried? Will donating change these relationships?

> I didn't tell a soul about my plan until after I had received the approval call. I didn't want my friends or family to go through the inevitable roller coaster of feelings unnecessarily if I wasn't approved or changed my mind. My family's responses ran the full spectrum. One of my daughters thought it was pretty cool; the other summarily forbade me to donate. My mother cried. But my most moving conversation had been with my sister Janet and Gary, my brother-in-law, the recipient of my kidney voucher. They worried about his advancing kidney disease but were also

concerned about me. My words rang shallow, "Why not?" I had pondered that question for months yet still couldn't articulate my commitment to this life saving act."

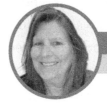

JUDY CHIASSON
Living Kidney Donor, 2019

> If you do not have family who is supportive of your decision, find friends who are supportive. You will need a group of people to support you physically, emotionally, and tangibly."

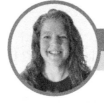

SARA GALLANDT
Living Kidney Donor, 2019

Expectations for Recognition

Do you have expectations as to how you should be treated after donation? Do you expect family, friends, or your community to recognize you as a hero? Are you seeking acceptance or notoriety?

> With time the initial kudos, attaboys, commendations, etc., will fade away. For everyone else, life will return to usual. You will need to adjust to this transition. So, try not to make judgments or have expectations. Just keep in mind that you DID something very extraordinary that less than one percent of the human race care to do. And to many you are a Human Angel!"

DAVE BORA
Living Kidney Donor, 1977
Kidney Recipient, 2018

Short and Long-Term Risks of Donation

Have you accepted the possible risks of surgery? Are you willing to accept any impact it could have? How would a recovery setback due to complications impact you and your family?

Anxiety and Fear

Are you a highly anxious person? Are you able to manage anxiety and fears well? Do you practice healthy ways to calm stress?

Relationship With Recipient

Do you expect donating will help or hinder the relationship with your recipient? Do you expect to develop a new relationship? How will you feel if your recipient does not want to meet you or does not express gratitude for your extraordinary gift?

> "The emotional part that you might not be aware of comes from the recipient. It is easier to give than receive. My recipient didn't know what to say or how to interact with me for quite a while. I just let it be and eventually we could talk about it."

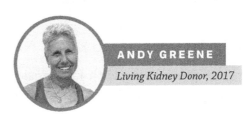

ANDY GREENE
Living Kidney Donor, 2017

> A unique dynamic can occur in kidney donation. A part of me was inside of a total stranger. Some donors and recipients form very close relationships; others never even meet. I heeded my coordinator's sage advice not to have any expectations, yet I was so happy that my recipient wanted to meet the

next day. We embraced tightly while our families looked on and cried. I was grateful to have the name and face of my kidney's new family. After that, we exchanged emails on our kidney-versaries, which felt like the right amount of contact for us."

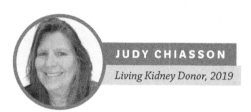

JUDY CHIASSON
Living Kidney Donor, 2019

Financial Concerns

Do you have a way to manage financially if you need to take extra time off from work or have unexpected medical expenses in the future? Have you considered the impact of taking time off work?

Mental Health

Have you been diagnosed with a mental illness, and if so, is it managed well or is it still a significant problem? Are you aware of the risks of depression after donation?

Life stressors

Are you dealing with family issues, divorce, a death, abuse, legal problems, or other major stressors?

Coping Strategies

What do you do when you are faced with difficult problems? Do you turn to alcohol or drugs? Do you have people or faith you turn to for help? How have you responded to hardship in the past?

WHAT EMOTIONS MIGHT I EXPECT TO FEEL?

> "My main concerns during the process had to do with the surgery and it actually working. Ultimately, this was out of my hands. The way I coped with this was by having good friends and family to talk with and process it through. I also spent a lot of time in prayer."

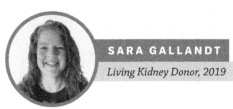

SARA GALLANDT
Living Kidney Donor, 2019

Motivation to Donate

Why are you considering donation? Do you feel a sense of duty? Are you looking for a purpose or to improve your quality of life?

> "My motivation was to help my whole family, take the burden of donation off my other siblings, and to improve my brother's quality of life. It was important to me that my brother knew that people love him enough to want to donate, even without him asking."

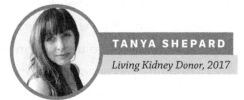

TANYA SHEPARD
Living Kidney Donor, 2017

Support for Caregiving

Do you have a caregiver to help during recovery? Do you have anyone to rely on if getting back to your normal responsibilities is delayed? Do you live with someone who can help with household chores, children, pets, and meals, as needed?

> A caregiver is vital. We could not have survived without our caregiver. My mom took care of us, she attended appointments and listened, she heard what we did not, she made sure we took meds, had meals ready, and got us up and walking even when we didn't want to."

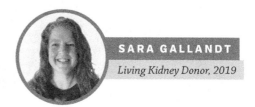

SARA GALLANDT
Living Kidney Donor, 2019

What can I do if I have difficult emotions?

The journey of organ donation is often full of intense emotions; recognizing that you're not alone in these emotions can help validate and accept them as they come. This acceptance may encourage you to feel your emotions without reacting in exaggerated or unhealthy ways. Reach out for support and comfort from others during this unique time. Engaging with others who have had similar experiences may allow you to see your situation from a realistic perspective rather than a dramatized version that can result when emotions are intense. Ask your donor team for recommendations to find transplant and donor support groups and mentors. These can often be found through medical centers, charitable foundations, churches, and online. You may also want to consider the benefits of a mental health professional during this time. After all, organ donation is truly a once-in-a-lifetime experience, so make the very best of it!

WHAT EMOTIONS MIGHT I EXPECT TO FEEL?

" I think the most important emotional aspect of donation is that you start to laugh with joy more and you live your life with more passion."

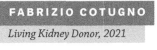

FABRIZIO COTUGNO
Living Kidney Donor, 2021

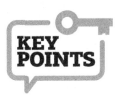

KEY POINTS

- Living kidney donation may be one of the most satisfying experiences in your life, but it may also be one of the most emotional.

- Being prepared for emotional highs and lows may help you recognize them as normal and work through them more easily.

- The psychosocial evaluation helps to identify any areas of concern that may lead to difficult emotions during or after donation.

- Keeping connected with trusted family, friends, a support group, or a mental health professional may help you to manage any complex emotions of living kidney donation.

CHAPTER TEN

How Do I Stay Healthy With One Kidney?

"*Share Your Spare*" has become a popular phrase for promoting living kidney donation. It's catchy and cute—and it works! But does it accurately represent what it means to donate a kidney? Do we really have a spare, like we have a spare tire in our car? Well, not exactly. Donating a kidney is much more complex and heroic than simply carrying around an extra part. *When we donate, we take on some risk, just like any other heroic act.*

We are born with a set number of nephrons, the tiny filtering units in our kidneys. We cannot grow more nephrons; if they die, we cannot regenerate them. The more healthy nephrons we have, the stronger our kidneys perform. When we donate a kidney, we forfeit half of them, leaving us with a single healthy kidney capable of picking up a portion of the lost workload. Over time, our kidneys age and both donors and non-donors alike experience a decline in kidney function. However, if you are approved to donate, your transplant team believes you will have enough kidney function to last your lifetime.

What you won't have is as much wiggle room. For that reason, it is essential to take care of your remaining kidney. A lifetime of healthy living, routine checkups, informing healthcare providers that you have one kidney, and following up on anything that does not seem right can help prevent any issues. If caught early, concerns can be addressed and bigger problems prevented.

By committing to preserving kidney function, you can minimize the risks of living with one kidney. In fact, your life after donation can be just as good, or even better, than before. Donors are courageous, generous, and self-sacrificing, and they can say:

"It isn't a spare. But I care. So I share!"

> I felt more connected with so many people. I had put myself out there to make a difference and felt good about taking an active role in life that was undeniably helpful. I also found out how healthy I was to be able to donate which inspired me to stay that way."

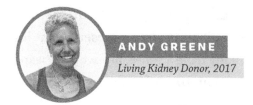

ANDY GREENE
Living Kidney Donor, 2017

Get Routine Kidney Checkups

Just because you feel well does not mean everything is fine inside. Many health conditions do not have symptoms in their early stages. As you have learned, kidney disease is one of them and can progress without symptoms until in its later stages. In addition, the primary conditions that cause kidney disease, like high blood pressure and high blood sugar, also typically do not have symptoms until they have progressed. For these reasons and more, you must see your healthcare provider for regular checkups, even when you feel healthy. These visits can help you avoid health problems in the future. It is a donor's responsibility to schedule these visits.

When selecting who manages your future care, keep in mind that not all healthcare providers have the same level of expertise in managing the health of a kidney donor. Find a provider who understands the potential impact of reduced kidney function on the body, the long-term risks associated with living kidney donation, and who will monitor for problems that can cause kidney damage. Before meeting with a provider, consider preparing for this discussion by refamiliarizing yourself with Chapter 2 on what kidneys do for the body and the ways they can become damaged. Although your routine care might be with a primary care provider, ensure they are willing to collaborate with a nephrologist or a transplant team if needed.

How often you need to see a healthcare provider for routine checkups depends on your overall health. A healthy kidney donor should schedule checkups at least once per year. If any health problems are detected, your healthcare provider may recommend more frequent visits for closer monitoring.

Not all providers include kidney function tests in routine physical exams. Therefore, confirm that these tests are completed. Sometimes donors are told that these tests do not apply to donors. However, they provide the best overall index for monitoring kidney function.[160] Keep track of your test results and look for trends over time. If your numbers worsen, seek help to prevent a problem. As you are now aware, the earlier issues are detected and treated, the better.

In the unlikely event that your test results indicate your kidney function is at the level of late-stage three or early-stage four kidney disease (eGFR less than 45), see a nephrologist[161] to help prevent further decline and address other problems that reduced kidney function can cause to the body.

"Make sure you have a doctor you are confident in with a breadth of understanding for what donors might encounter. This is important for protecting your kidney health."

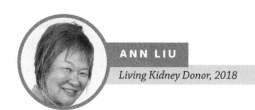

ANN LIU

Living Kidney Donor, 2018

Maintain a Healthy Weight

Maintaining a healthy weight is essential for kidney health. Being overweight or obese can lead to kidney damage because excess weight puts extra strain on the kidneys, forcing them to work harder and filter more waste than normal. This additional workload can cause damage to the kidneys over time. In addition, carrying too much fat can compress and put pressure on the kidneys. People who are overweight are also more likely to have high blood pressure and blood sugar problems.[162]

In addition to a sensible diet, regular physical activity can boost your metabolism, which means your body will be better at burning calories, even when resting. A faster metabolism can help you maintain a healthy weight and lower your risk of developing conditions known to cause kidney damage.[163]

Living donors who are obese have increased surgical risks and increased risk of kidney failure after donation.[164] Transplant centers often require people who are overweight to lose weight before donation to reduce these risks. However, it is not uncommon for donors to gain those pounds back.[165] If required to lose weight before donation, it is important to maintain the weight loss to protect your kidney function.

Be Heart Healthy

Since the heart and kidneys work together to maintain good health and rely on each other to function correctly, when one has a problem, the other is affected. When the kidneys are not filtering sufficiently, they are less able to control blood pressure, clean the blood as well as they should, and remove extra fluid. As a result, the heart needs to pump harder to get blood through the kidneys, putting extra stress on the heart. This extra strain can lead to heart disease.[166] Consequently, if the heart is not functioning sufficiently, it may not be able to supply the kidneys with enough blood, which can cause kidney damage.[167] Therefore, it is important to care for both the heart and kidneys to maintain good overall health.

How do I keep my heart healthy?

Keeping your heart healthy may be achieved by making good lifestyle choices, such as maintaining healthy blood pressure, avoiding excess salt, eating a heart-healthy diet, and getting plenty of exercise.

Maintain healthy blood pressure. Work with a healthcare provider to set a blood pressure goal that is appropriate for you and make lifestyle choices that help maintain it. If you have problems with blood pressure, checking your blood pressure once a year at a routine physical exam may not be enough. In this case, it is a good idea to keep a blood pressure monitor at home and know how to use it correctly. Also, follow any blood pressure medication recommendations from your provider.[168]

Avoid excess salt. Sodium, a mineral found in salt, is essential for balancing water and minerals in the body but consuming too much salt can cause kidney problems.[169] When you have too much salt in your diet, your body retains extra water to dilute the excess sodium. This puts a strain on your kidneys, which work to remove this extra water. The increased volume of water also puts extra pressure on your blood vessels, causing them to stiffen and narrow, and on your heart, leading to high blood pressure and added kidney stress.

Eat a heart-healthy diet. A heart-healthy diet involves choosing foods that are low in saturated animal fats, processed fats, sodium, and sugar, but are high in nutrients such as fiber, vitamins, and minerals. Heart-healthy foods include whole grains, fresh produce, legumes, and healthy fats such as olive oil, avocado, nuts, and seeds.[170]

Commit to regular physical activity. Exercise strengthens the heart and improves its efficiency at pumping blood. This can help to lower blood pressure and reduce the workload on your kidneys.[171]

Eat a Kidney-Healthy Diet

Maintaining a healthy diet is crucial for kidney health, as kidneys filter everything that enters the body. To eat in a way that supports kidney health, focus on whole, natural foods, and pay attention to the right amount and type of protein. If you are unsure how to eat a kidney-healthy diet, consider consulting with a doctor or registered dietitian who specializes in renal diets to create a personalized plan.

Focus on Whole, Natural Foods

For those without kidney disease, following a kidney-healthy diet does not require following a specific eating regimen. Instead, it simply means eating whole, natural foods and avoiding processed, inflammatory foods.[172] This involves making most of your diet consist of nutrient-dense vegetables, fruits, whole grains, nuts, seeds, and healthy fats. It also means avoiding inflammatory foods and ingredients like artificial food additives, manufactured foods, processed fats, processed meats, and high glycemic ingredients like sugar and white flour.

> I always wanted to be healthy, but I wasn't. I was 40 and had never touched a vegetable, was overweight, and hurting constantly. Then I was called to donate. If the Holy Spirit tells me to donate a kidney, I'm going to donate a kidney. I

knew people donated kidneys and I could donate one if mine were healthy enough. So, I decided to get healthy by doing small things at a time. I started with one vegetable and went from there eating anti-inflammatory plant-based foods. It improved every area of my health and I felt like I was 20 again. Once you start to feel better, you want to continue. If you value your life, you will give some things up.

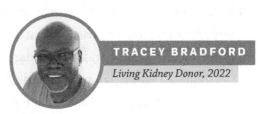

TRACEY BRADFORD
Living Kidney Donor, 2022

Focus on the Right Amount and Type of Protein

Eating protein is essential, but it is important to exercise caution when selecting the amount and type of protein you consume on a regular basis.

Avoid consuming excess protein. Protein is essential for functions like building muscle, repairing tissue, making new cells, and fighting infections. But the amount of protein you need depends on factors like your weight, overall health, and activity level. Many adults consume more protein than they need, leading to problems. When protein is consumed, waste is produced that the kidneys must remove from the body, making them work harder. This additional strain can cause kidney injury.[173,174,175] Before starting a long-term high-protein diet or protein supplementation, speak with a healthcare provider to determine if it is safe for you.

Choose more plant protein sources. In addition to avoiding excess protein, choosing healthy protein sources is also important for protecting your kidney health. Protein can come from both plant and animal sources. Animal proteins, such as beef, poultry, fish, and dairy, are considered "complete" because they provide the essential amino acids needed to make the proteins the body needs. However, animal proteins produce acid and increase ammonia production, which can put extra pressure on the kidneys and damage sensitive kidney cells.[176,177,178]

On the other hand, plant proteins, such as beans, lentils, soy, nuts, and whole grains, can provide protein while causing less stress on the kidneys.[179] Additionally, these plant proteins offer nutrients like fiber, vitamins, minerals, and antioxidants. However, plant proteins do not provide all essential amino acids, so it is important to eat a variety of plant proteins to get all the amino acids you need. To note, people with advanced stages of chronic kidney disease may need to avoid specific plant proteins containing high phosphorus and potassium levels.

Eating protein from a variety of plant sources and minimizing animal sources is helpful in protecting the kidneys from damage that may be caused by animal protein.[180]

Control Blood Sugar

Elevated blood sugar can cause damage to the blood vessels in the kidneys, leading to weakened vessels that are prone to blockages. This can restrict the flow of blood to the kidneys and cause their filtering nephrons to die.[181] About 40% of American adults have prediabetes or diabetes, which means their blood sugar levels are high enough to harm the body.[182,183] Even if you do not have diabetes, too much sugar in your blood can lead to insulin resistance, a precursor to type-2 diabetes, and kidney damage.[184]

To monitor your blood sugar and ensure that your average blood sugar is not creeping up over time, get an A1C test at least yearly.[185] An A1C is a blood test that checks the average blood sugar level over the past three months.

- Normal: below 5.7%
- Prediabetes: between 5.7% and 6.4%
- Diabetes: 6.5% or higher

How do I keep my blood sugar level healthy?

Maintaining a healthy weight, exercising on a regular basis, and making wise food choices can help avoid elevated blood sugar levels and its damaging effects.

Avoid weight gain. Carrying excess fat, especially around the middle, can lead to chronic inflammation. Chronic inflammation is a risk factor for developing type-2 diabetes.[186]

Stay physically active. Vigorous movement can improve your body's sensitivity to insulin, which helps keep your blood sugar levels within a healthy range.[187]

Choose high-fiber foods. Plant foods high in fiber slows food absorption after eating, promotes feeling full, reduces cravings, and prevents overeating. Good sources of soluble fiber include whole grains, high-fiber fruits and vegetables, legumes, and nuts.[188]

Focus on low-glycemic foods. High-glycemic foods are absorbed quickly and cause a rapid increase in blood sugar. Choosing low-glycemic foods helps to avoid these sudden spikes.[189,190] Focus on low-glycemic foods such as beans, lentils, nuts, whole grains, non-starchy vegetables, and healthy fats. Avoid high-glycemic foods like sugar, white flour, potatoes, and white rice. Eating healthy fats and proteins alongside foods that can raise blood sugar may also help to slow your food digestion and absorption and help prevent spikes in blood sugar.

Stay Hydrated

Every part of the body needs water to function. When you lose more water than you consume, your body becomes dehydrated, meaning it does not have enough water to work properly.

Kidneys like to be hydrated. Drinking plenty of fluids helps them to perform their work. Without enough water, problems can result, such as kidney stones, reduced blood flow to the kidneys, urinary tract infections,[191] and clogged kidneys.[192]

We are at the greatest risk of dehydration when we lose more water than usual, such as in hot or dry climates, when exercising, sweating excessively, drinking alcohol heavily, taking laxatives, or when sick and vomiting or have diarrhea. Although, simply not drinking enough water can cause dehydration too. Signs of mild dehydration include:[193]

- Feeling very thirsty
- Dry mouth
- Feeling tired
- Dizziness
- Dark urine
- Urine that smells strong

How much fluid should I drink?

There is no specific number to indicate how much fluid you need to stay hydrated. The amount of water you need varies depending on factors like your activity level, climate, health, and diet. Thirst is generally a good indicator of when you need to drink more water. As a general guide, adults should aim for daily fluid intake of about:

- 125 ounces (16 cups or 3.7 liters) a day for men
- 91 ounces (11 cups or 2.7 liters) a day for women[194,195]

Not all fluids need to come from water or beverages. Some fruits and vegetables contain a good amount of water that also counts towards your daily fluid intake.

Limit Alcohol

Drinking a little alcohol now and then is generally not a problem. Drinking too much, however, can cause serious problems.[196] Excessive alcohol consumption can lead to high blood pressure,[197] dehydration,[198] and liver disease—all of which can cause damage to the kidneys.

The amount of alcohol that is considered too much varies depending on factors such as gender, age, and weight. As a general rule, moderation is recommended. The National Institute of Diabetes and Digestive and Kidney Diseases (NIDDKD) indicates that moderation means men should limit their alcohol intake to one to two drinks per day, while women and people over 65 should limit their intake to one drink per day. One drink is considered:

- 12 ounces of beer
- 5 ounces of wine
- 1.5 ounces of liquor[199]

Heavy drinking, averaging more than four drinks per day for men and more than three drinks per day for women, can double the risk of developing kidney disease.[200] Consult with a healthcare provider to determine the safe amount of alcohol for you.

Get Plenty of Safe Exercise

We all know that exercise is essential for good health. And you have learned that exercise is particularly good for kidney health because it can assist in managing weight, maintain a healthy heart, control blood pressure, and help regulate blood sugar levels. However, you may not know how much exercise is needed to gain these benefits and how much is too much.

How much should I exercise?

The amount of activity right for you can vary depending on your age, weight, health, and fitness level. In general, it is recommended that adults get at least 150 minutes of moderate-intensity aerobic activity or 75 minutes of vigorous-intensity aerobic exercise per week. It is also recommended to do muscle-strengthening activities like lifting weights or calisthenics at least two days per week.[201]

While these guidelines are a good starting point, they may not be appropriate for everyone. It is best to talk to a healthcare provider before starting an exercise program.

How much exercise is too much?

Overexertion occurs when you put too much physical strain on your body, causing muscle tissue to breakdown, leading to a release of waste products in the bloodstream. This can lead to a range of health problems, including kidney damage. People who participate in endurance sports like marathons and those who do high-intensity training have a higher risk of overexertion. Listen to your body's warning signals and avoid pushing too hard to protect your kidneys from problems caused by overexertion.

Stay hydrated. Drinking plenty of fluids before, during, and after exercise, especially water, keeps your body hydrated and your muscles working properly.

Warm up. Warming your muscles before you exercise gradually increases your heart rate and blood flow and prepares your muscles for exercise.

Listen to your body. Paying attention to your body's warning signs and resting if you feel pain or fatigue allows you to recover and prevent muscle tissue breakdown.

"My health is great, but I take care of myself because I want to protect my only kidney left."

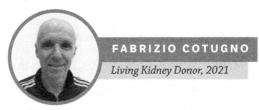
FABRIZIO COTUGNO
Living Kidney Donor, 2021

Avoid Injuries

The ribs and back muscles help to protect the kidneys from injury, but they can still be damaged by a strong blow to the abdomen or back. This type of trauma to the kidneys can damage their delicate filters, which is why it is important to take precautions to protect them. To reduce the risk of injury, doctors often advise kidney donors to avoid contact sports such as football, soccer, hockey, boxing, martial arts, and wrestling. Sometimes doctors may instead recommend wearing extra protective padding, but this will not eliminate the risk. If your back receives a forceful hit, especially if you see blood in your urine, it is important to schedule a checkup with your healthcare provider.

Take Medication and Supplement Precautions

All medications and supplements pass through the kidneys in some form[202] and can potentially cause harm if not taken with proper precautions. To help prevent problems, it is important to know your kidney function test results and share them with prescribing healthcare providers. It is also a good idea to keep a current list of all medications and supplements you are taking and be prepared to ask questions about their safety and potential interactions with other substances. Educating yourself about medication and supplement safety can go a long way in safeguarding your kidneys.

Over-the-Counter Medications

Over-the-counter (OTC) medications are often perceived as safe because they do not require a prescription. However, this is not always the case. Long-term use of certain OTC medications can damage the kidneys and even cause kidney failure. It is essential to be aware of the risks and use these medications only as directed and for a minimal duration, if at all.

Try to avoid nonsteroidal anti-inflammatory drugs (NSAIDs). NSAIDs are used to reduce pain, inflammation, and fevers. They are sold alone or in medications labeled for colds, coughs, and sleeping problems. However, regular use of NSAIDs can reduce blood flow to the kidneys and causes them harm.[203] Therefore, they should only be taken for less than ten days,[204] at the lowest possible doses, no higher than the label instructs, and for the shortest time.[205] Those with reduced kidney function should avoid them altogether without a recommendation from their healthcare provider.

Use aspirin cautiously. Aspirin, also a NSAID, when taken as directed on the label for occasional pain, does not seem to increase the risk of kidney disease in people with normal kidney function. However, if you take buffered aspirin for conditions like arthritis that require multiple daily doses over extended periods, it is important to talk to your healthcare provider first.[206]

Prescription Medications

Certain prescription medications can harm the kidneys, even when taken in small amounts or only occasionally. That's why it is essential to tell all prescribing healthcare providers your kidney status. If your kidney function is not within a normal range, your provider can take caution when choosing medications and dosages to reduce the risk of harm.[207]

Take caution with antimicrobials. Antimicrobials are important drugs used to treat infections caused by microorganisms, such as bacteria, viruses, and fungi. These medications include antibiotics, antifungals, and antivirals. Certain antimicrobial medications need to be taken in smaller doses or avoided when kidney function is reduced.[208]

Take caution with cholesterol medications. Statins are medications often prescribed to help lower cholesterol levels. Maintaining healthy cholesterol levels is important for heart and kidney health. However, if your kidney function is not within normal range, your provider may need to adjust your dosage to protect your kidney.[209]

Take caution with contrast dye. Imaging tests like MRIs, CT scans, and angiograms help diagnose diseases and injuries. Sometimes, a contrast dye is used to make the image clearer. However, this dye may cause problems with kidneys particularly in those with advanced kidney disease (GFR below 30).[210] In this case, talk to your healthcare provider about using as little as possible and drink plenty of water before and after the test to help protect your kidney.

Take caution with prescription laxatives. Laxatives are medications used to treat constipation. In general, OTC laxatives are safe for most people, but some prescription laxatives used for cleaning the bowel, usually before a colonoscopy, can harm the kidneys. It is important to avoid laxatives with high magnesium sulfate or sodium phosphate concentrations,[211] and instead to use bowel cleansers that contain polyethylene glycol mixed with salts and water.[212]

Nutritional Supplements

Taking supplements is a common practice, but the risks of doing so are often overlooked. Like medications, supplements pass through the kidneys and can cause harm to them, either because they contain harmful ingredients or because the kidneys cannot effectively clear out the waste.[213] Additionally, supplements can interact with other supplements or medications. Avoid using supplements without consulting a healthcare provider to ensure the safety of any supplement regimen.[214]

Recreational Drugs

Using street drugs, such as cocaine, heroin, and amphetamines, can have dangerous and potentially fatal consequences. These drugs can cause high blood pressure, stroke, heart failure, and they can also cause kidney damage.[215,216] The effect of marijuana on kidney health is not entirely clear. However, according to limited research, marijuana use might not affect healthy kidneys but may cause a more rapid decline in kidney function in those with chronic kidney disease.[217,218]

Do Not Smoke

Smoking is known to harm nearly every organ of the body,[219] so it is no surprise that smoking is harmful to the kidneys. Smoking can reduce blood flow, narrow the blood vessels in the kidneys, and cause their arteries to become thickened and hardened. Furthermore, these effects can increase blood pressure and heart rate and cause inflammation and oxidative stress.[220]

Manage Stress

Stress is a normal part of life that occurs when something disrupts the balance of your mind and body. Stress can be emotional, such as anxiety, loneliness, anger, or depression. It can also be physical, like infections, injuries, surgeries, or diseases.[221] When your body experiences stress, it reacts with physical changes, known as the "fight or flight" response, which can include increased blood pressure, a faster heart rate, increases in fat and sugar in the blood, and inflammation. These reactions are normal and purposeful, but they can become problems if your body is reacting to stress for too long. Chronic stress can lead to conditions like high blood pressure and high blood sugar.[222] Therefore, managing stress is important for preventing kidney damage.[223] While you may always have some level of stress, taking steps to help calm your body's response to stress can help avoid the health problems it can cause.

Incorporate simple strategies to help calm your stress response throughout the day, such as:

- Slow deep breathing
- Prayer and meditation
- Physical activity
- Stretching
- Social connection
- Hobbies
- Positive thinking
- Playing music

Taking care of your kidney after donation entails making choices that promote its health. Donors are real-life heroes for prioritizing the well-being of others. But remember, it is equally important to be a hero for your own body! By making small sacrifices, you can keep your kidney functioning at its best and enjoy a lifetime of good health.

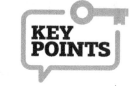

KEY POINTS

- Kidney donors have less "extra" kidney function, making it especially important to preserve kidney nephrons.

- Routine kidney checkups are important for detecting and addressing any issues early on to prevent bigger problems from developing in the future.

- With continued commitment to health, life after donation is typically the same as before donation—or better!

Donor Resources

Alliance for Paired Kidney Donation
paireddonation.org
admin@paireddonation.org
(419) 740-5249

Provides support on all aspects of paired kidney donation. The APKD uses an algorithm to match one incompatible pair with another to find the best possible match and significantly reduce the wait time for a kidney transplant.

Alport Syndrome Foundation
alportsyndome.org
info@alportsyndome.org
(480) 800-3510

A non-profit led by Alport syndrome patients with the mission to improve the lives of people living with Alport syndrome through education, empowerment, and advocacy.

American Foundation for Donation and Transplantation
afdt.org
skinner@afdt.org
(804) 323-9893

Maintains the Living Organ Donor Network, which provides optional life, disability, and medical insurance for financial protection in the event complications are experienced as a result of a kidney donation for a one-time fee.

American Kidney Fund
kidneyfund.org
(800) 795-3226

Assists donors with out-of-pocket expenses related to their kidney donation with the Safety Net Grant Program, often including the cost of travel and lodging or lost wages during the transplant process.

American Living Organ Donor Fund
helplivingdonorssavelives.org
info@alodf.org
(215) 601-6530

Helps organ donors with non-medical expenses related to organ donation, including travel, lodging, lost wages, and other costs of donation and recovery. No financial criteria are necessary to apply. They also provide a comprehensive list for state specific resources on their website, helplivingdonorssavelives.org.

American Transplant Foundation
americantransplantfoundation.org
(303) 757-0959

Offers a Patient Assistance Program to help living donors with significant financial hardships due to lost wages to help pay for essential living expenses, such as mortgages or rent.

Donate Life America
donatelife.net

Launched the National Donate Life Living Donor Registry, a national registry for prospective living donors. People between the ages of 18-

65 who register their decision to be a deceased organ, eye and tissue donor through the National Donate Life Registry, RegisterMe.org, will also be offered the opportunity to register their interest in being a living kidney donor.

Kidney Transplant Centers
kidneytransplantcenters.org

Compares the performance and services of all kidney transplant centers in the United States, provided by the National Kidney Registry.

Living Donors Online
livingdonorsonline.org

An online community for living donor education, support, and advocacy. Living Donor Buddies is a program administered by Living Donors Online that matches potential living donors with people who have previously donated for support.

National Foundation for Transplants
transplants.org
info@transplants.org
(901) 684-1697

Assists living donors in fundraising to cover lost wages, travel, food, lodging, medications, childcare and other expenses related to donation.

National Kidney Foundation
kidney.org
(855) 653-2273

NKF is a leading pioneer of scientific research and accelerating change. They also provide support and extensive education to people with kidney disease and to living kidney donors. NKF Peers connects kidney patients with trained mentors who have been there themselves.

National Kidney Registry (NKR)
kidneyregistry.org
donor-shield.org

Helps to increase the number of kidney transplants from living donors by improving donor-recipient matches, manages voucher programs, and offers protection and support to living kidney donors. Donors who participate in a National Kidney Registry Swap, Voucher Program, Paired Exchange Program, or donate through a Donor Shield Direct Center are eligible for the Donor Shield financial protection program. Benefits include lost wage reimbursement, travel and lodging expenses, legal support, complication protection, home blood draws, and more.

National Living Donor Assistance Center
livingdonorassistance.org
NLDAC@livingdonorassistance.org
(888) 870-5002

A national organization funded by a federal government grant helps donors with non-medical expenses related to donation, including travel expenses, lost wages, and dependent care expenses for people being evaluated for or undergoing living organ donation that cannot be paid by their recipient, a state program, or an insurance company. Eligibility is based on the transplant recipient's household income.

NFK CARES

nkfcares@kidney.org
(855) 653-2273

Speak with an English or Spanish-speaking trained specialist who will answer your questions and listen to your concerns. Designed for patients, living donors, family members, and care partners.

NKF PEERS

NKFpeers@kidney.org
(855) 653-7337

Speak with a trained peer mentor who can answer your questions and share their living donation experiences with you. A social worker will help connect you with a PEER who is right for you.

Organ Procurement and Transplant Network (OPTN)

optn.transplant.hrsa.gov
(888) 894-6361

Helps to increase the number of transplants, provide equal access to transplants, improve transplant and donor outcomes, and promote living donor and recipient safety. Operates a national kidney paired donation (KPD) system.

United Network for Organ Sharing (UNOS)
transplantliving.org
unos.org
(888) 894-6361

The private, non-profit organization that manages the U.S organ transplant system under contract with the federal government.

Southwest Airlines
southwest.com

Offers free airfare for medical transportation of patients at qualifying transplant centers. For a list of qualifying centers, visit: southwest.com/html/southwest-difference/community-involvement/charities/medical_transportation.html.

Transplant Recipients International Organization
trioweb.org
(813) 800-8746

Teams with United Airlines to provide free airfare for living donors, recipients, caregivers, and candidates for transplant-related travel.

References & Additional Reading

1   Chronic Kidney Disease in the United States, 2021. Centers for Disease Control and Prevention. https://www.cdc.gov/kidneydisease/publications-resources/ckd-national-facts.html. Accessed February 2022.

2   Chronic Kidney Disease Basics. Centers for Disease Control and Prevention. https://www.cdc.gov/kidneydisease/basics.html. Updated February 28, 2022. Accessed March 2022.

3   The Top 10 Causes of Death. World Health Organization. https://www.who.int/news-room/fact-sheets/detail/the-top-10-causes-of-death. Published December 2020. Accessed July 2022.

4   Chronic Kidney Disease Basics. Centers for Disease Control and Prevention. https://www.cdc.gov/kidneydisease/basics.html. Updated February 28, 2022. Accessed March 2022.

5   Data. Organ Procurement & Transplantation Network. U.S. Department of Health and Human Services. https://optn.transplant.hrsa.gov/data/

6   The Kidney Transplant Waitlist – What You Need to Know. National Kidney Foundation. https://www.kidney.org/atoz/content/transplant-waitlist. Accessed March 2022.

7   Choosing a Treatment for Kidney Failure. National Institute of Diabetes and Digestive and Kidney Diseases. https://www.niddk.nih.gov/health-information/kidney-disease/kidney-failure/choosing-treatment Updated January 2018. Accessed September 2022.

8   A Proclamation on National Donate Life Month. The White House. https://www.whitehouse.gov/briefing-room/presidential-actions/2022/03/31/a-proclamation-on-national-donate-life-month-2022/. Published March 31, 2022. Accessed April 2022.

9   Living Donation. United Network for Organ Sharing. https://unos.org/transplant/living-donation/. Accessed March 2022.

10   Slevin J, Taylor A. Understanding what the public know about their kidneys and what they do: Findings from Ipsos MORI survey 2014. Think Kidneys. National Health Service. https://www.thinkkidneys.nhs.uk/aki/wp-content/uploads/2015/01/Think-Kidneys-Report-270115-Understanding-what-the-public-know-about-their-kidneys-and-what-they-do.pdf. Published January 15, 2015.

11   Slevin J, Taylor A. Understanding what the public know about their kidneys and what they do: Findings from Ipsos MORI survey 2014. Think Kidneys. National Health Service. https://www.thinkkidneys.nhs.uk/aki/wp-content/uploads/2015/01/Think-Kidneys-Report-270115-Understanding. Published January 15, 2015.

12   Berns J. Patient education: Chronic kidney disease (Beyond the Basics). *UpToDate*. July 8, 2021. https://www.uptodate.com/contents/chronic-kidney-disease-beyond-the-basics

13   Slevin J, Taylor A. Understanding what the public know about their kidneys and what they do: Findings from Ipsos MORI survey 2014. Think Kidneys. National Health Service. https://www.thinkkidneys.nhs.uk/aki/wp-content/uploads/2015/01/Think-Kidneys-Report-270115-Understanding. Published January 15, 2015.

14   Mineral & Bone Disorder in Chronic Kidney Disease. National Institute of Diabetes and Digestive and Kidney Diseases. https://www.niddk.nih.gov/health-information/kidney-disease/mineral-bone-disorder. Updated November 2021.

15   Fluid and Electrolyte Balance. Medline Plus. National Library of Medicine. https://medlineplus.gov/fluidandelectrolytebalance.html. Accessed February 2021.

16   Metabolic Acidosis. National Kidney Foundation. https://www.kidney.org/atoz/content/metabolic-acidosis. Accessed March 2021.

17   Your Kidneys & How They Work. National Institute of Diabetes and Digestive and Kidney Diseases. https://www.niddk.nih.gov/health-information/kidney-disease/kidneys-how-they-work. Published June 2018.

18   Mineral & Bone Disorder in Chronic Kidney Disease.National Institute of Diabetes and Digestive and Kidney Diseases. https://www.niddk.nih.gov/health-information/kidney-disease/mineral-bone-disorder. Updated November 2021.

19   5 Drugs You May Need to Avoid or Adjust if You Have Kidney Disease. National Kidney Foundation. https://www.kidney.org/atoz/content/5-drugs-you-may-need-to-avoid-or-adjust-if-you-have-kidney-disease. Accessed March 2022.

20   Your Kidneys & How They Work. National Institute of Diabetes and Digestive and Kidney Diseases. https://www.niddk.nih.gov/health-information/kidney-disease/kidneys-how-they-work. Updated June 2018.

21   Acute Kidney Injury (AKI). National Kidney Foundation. https://www.kidney.org/atoz/content/AcuteKidneyInjury. Accessed June 2022.

22   Rastogi A. Kidney Disease: What You Should Know. YouTube. https://www.youtube.com/watch?v=W0OmgjNRSIE. Published August 24, 2018.

23   Coca S, Singanamala S, Parikh C. Chronic kidney disease after acute kidney injury: a systematic review and meta-analysis. *Kidney International.* March 1, 2012. 81(5):442-448. doi: 10.1038/ki.2011.379

24   Heung M, Chawla L. Acute Kidney Injury: Gateway to Chronic Kidney Disease. *Nephron Clinical Practice*. September 2014. 127:30-34. doi: 10.1159/000363675

25   Chronic kidney disease (CKD). National Kidney Foundation. https://www.kidney.org/atoz/content/about-chronic-kidney-disease#what-are-symptoms. Accessed June 2022

26   Rastogi A. Kidney Disease: What You Should Know. YouTube. https://www.youtube.com/watch?v=W0OmgjNRSIE. Published August 24, 2018.

27   Rastogi A. Kidney Disease: What You Should Know. YouTube. https://www.youtube.com/watch?v=W0OmgjNRSIE. Published August 24, 2018.

28   Symptoms & Causes of Diabetes. National Institute of Diabetes and Digestive and Kidney Diseases. https://www.niddk.nih.gov/health-information/diabetes/overview/symptoms-causes. Updated December 2016. Accessed June 2022.

29   Diabetes and Chronic Kidney Disease. Centers for Disease Control and Prevention. https://www.cdc.gov/diabetes/managing/diabetes-kidney-disease.html#:~:text=Each%20kidney%20is%20made%20up,which%20can%20damage%20kidneys%20too. Updated May 7, 2021. Accessed June 2022.

30   Diabetes and Chronic Kidney Disease. Centers for Disease Control and Prevention. https://www.cdc.gov/diabetes/managing/diabetes-kidney-disease.html#:~:text=Each%20kidney%20is%20made%20up,which%20can%20damage%20kidneys%20too. Updated May 7, 2021. Accessed June 2022.

31   How High Blood Pressure Can Lead to Kidney Damage or Failure. American Heart Association. https://www.heart.org/en/health-topics/high-blood-pressure/health-threats-from-high-blood-pressure/how-high-blood-pressure-can-lead-to-kidney-damage-or-failure. Updated March 4, 2022. Accessed June 2022.

32   High Blood Pressure & Kidney Disease. National Institute of Diabetes and Digestive and Kidney Diseases. https://www.niddk.nih.gov/health-information/kidney-disease/high-blood-pressure. Updated March 2020. Accessed June 2022.

33   High Blood Pressure & Kidney Disease. National Institute of Diabetes and Digestive and Kidney Diseases. https://www.niddk.nih.gov/health-information/kidney-disease/high-blood-pressure. Updated March 2020. Accessed June 2022.

34   High Blood Pressure & Kidney Disease. National Institute of Diabetes and Digestive and Kidney Diseases. https://www.niddk.nih.gov/health-information/kidney-disease/high-blood-pressure. Updated March 2020. Accessed June 2022.

35   Heart Disease & Kidney Disease. National Institute of Diabetes and Digestive and Kidney Diseases. https://www.niddk.nih.gov/health-information/kidney-disease/heart-disease. Updated June 2016. Accessed June 2022.

36   How High Blood Pressure Can Lead to Kidney Damage or Failure. American Heart Association. https://www.heart.org/en/health-topics/high-blood-pressure/health-threats-from-high-blood-pressure/how-high-blood-pressure-can-lead-to-kidney-damage-or-failure. Updated March 4, 2022. Accessed June 2022.

37   Inherited Kidney Diseases. National Kidney Foundation. https://www.kidney.org/atoz/content/inherited-kidney-disease. Accessed July 2022.

38   Rastogi A. Kidney Disease: What You Should Know. YouTube. https://www.youtube.com/watch?v=W0OmgjNRSIE. Published August 24, 2018.

39   Symptoms & Causes of Kidney Infection (Pyelonephritis). National Institute of Diabetes and Digestive and Kidney Diseases. https://www.niddk.nih.gov/health-information/urologic-diseases/kidney-infection-pyelonephritis/symptoms-causes. Updated April 2017. Accessed July 2022.

40   Duke University. COVID-19 can directly infect and damage human kidney cells. ScienceDaily. www.sciencedaily.com/releases/2022/04/220421181201.htm. Published April 21, 2022.

41   Lupus and Kidney Disease. National Institute of Diabetes and Digestive and Kidney Diseases. https://www.niddk.nih.gov/health-information/kidney-disease/lupus-nephritis. Updated January 2017. Accessed March 2022.

42	Preminger G. Urinary Tract Obstruction. Merck Manual. https://www.merckmanuals.com/home/kidney-and-urinary-tract-disorders/obstruction-of-the-urinary-tract/urinary-tract-obstruction. Updated September 2022. Accessed February 2023.

43	Dunkler D, Dehghan M, Teo K, Heinze G, Gao P, Kohl M. Diet and kidney disease in high-risk individuals with type 2 diabetes mellitus. *JAMA Intern Med*. 2013;173(18):1682-92. doi: 10.1001/jamainternmed.2013.9051

44	Akchurin O, Kaskel F. Update on inflammation in Chronic Kidney Disease. *Blood Purif*. 2015;39:84-92. doi: 10.1159/000368940

45	Which Drugs are Harmful to Your Kidneys? National Kidney Foundation. https://www.kidney.org/atoz/content/drugs-your-kidneys. Accessed March 2022.

46	Haroun M, Jaar B, Hoffman S, Comstock G, George W, Klag M, et al. Risk Factors for Chronic Kidney Disease: A Prospective Study of 23,534 Men and Women in Washington County, Maryland. *JASN*. 2003;14(11):2934-2941. doi: 10.1097/01.ASN.0000095249.99803.85

47	Chronic Kidney Disease Surveillance System. Adults With Early-Stage Chronic Kidney Disease Are More Likely To Currently Smoke. Centers for Disease Control and Prevention. https://nccd.cdc.gov/CKD/AreYouAware.aspx?emailDate=March_2021. Updated March 2021. Accessed March 2022.

48	National Kidney Foundation. Can Dehydration Affect Your Kidneys? https://www.kidney.org/newsletter/can-dehydration-affect-your-kidneys. Published April 2018. Accessed March 2022.

49	Stress and Your Kidneys. National Kidney Foundation. https://www.kidney.org/atoz/content/Stress_and_your_Kidneys. Accessed March 2022.

50	Kidney Disease: The Basics. National Kidney Foundation. https://www.kidney.org/news/newsroom/fsindex. Accessed February 2022.

51	Chronic kidney disease (CKD). National Kidney Foundation. https://www.kidney.org/atoz/content/about-chronic-kidney-disease#what-are-symptoms. Accessed February 2022.

52	High Blood Pressure & Kidney Disease. National Institute of Diabetes and Digestive and Kidney Diseases. https://www.niddk.nih.gov/health-information/kidney-disease/high-blood-pressure. Updated March 2021. Accessed June 2022.

53	Rastogi A. Kidney Disease: What You Should Know. YouTube. https://www.youtube.com/watch?v=W0OmgjNRSIE. Published August 2018.

54	National Kidney Foundation. Quick Reference Guide on Kidney Disease Screening. https://www.kidney.org/kidneydisease/siemens_hcp_quickreference

55	National Kidney Foundation. Know your Kidney Numbers: Two Simple Tests. https://www.kidney.org/atoz/content/know-your-kidney-numbers-two-simple-tests

56	National Institute of Diabetes and Digestive and Kidney Diseases. Chronic Kidney Disease Tests & Diagnosis. October 2016. https://www.niddk.nih.gov/health-information/kidney-disease/chronic-kidney-disease-ckd/tests-diagnosis

57	Rastogi A. Kidney Disease: What You Should Know. YouTube. https://www.youtube.com/watch?v=W0OmgjNRSIE. Published August 2018.

58   National Institute of Diabetes and Digestive and Kidney Diseases. What is Kidney Failure? January 2018. https://www.niddk.nih.gov/health-information/kidney-disease/kidney-failure/what-is-kidney-failure

59   Berns J. Patient education: Chronic kidney disease (Beyond the Basics). *UpToDate*. 2021. https://www.uptodate.com/contents/chronic-kidney-disease-beyond-the-basics

60   National Kidney Foundation. Kidney Failure Risk Factor: Estimated Glomerular Filtration Rate (eGFR). https://www.kidney.org/content/kidney-failure-risk-factor-estimated-glomerular-filtration-rate-egfr

61   Rastogi A. Kidney Disease: What You Should Know. YouTube. https://www.youtube.com/watch?v=W0OmgjNRSIE. Published August 2018.

62   National Kidney Foundation. Kidney Disease: The Basics. https://www.kidney.org/news/newsroom/fsindex

63   Rastogi A. Kidney Disease: What You Should Know. YouTube. https://www.youtube.com/watch?v=W0OmgjNRSIE. Published August 2018.

64   Rastogi A. Kidney Disease: What You Should Know. YouTube. https://www.youtube.com/watch?v=W0OmgjNRSIE. Published August 2018.

65   About the CKD Initiative. Centers for Disease Control and Prevention. https://www.cdc.gov/kidneydisease/about-the-ckd-initiative.html. Published July 2022.

66   National Institute of Diabetes and Digestive and Kidney Diseases. Kidney Disease Statistics for the United States. https://www.niddk.nih.gov/health-information/health-statistics/kidney-disease. Updated September 2021.

67   Dialysis. National Kidney Foundation. https://www.kidney.org/atoz/content/dialysisinfo. Accessed July 2022.

68   Dialysis. National Kidney Foundation. https://www.kidney.org/atoz/content/dialysisinfo. Accessed July 2022.

69   Noone A, Pfeiffer R, Dorgan J, et al. Cancer-attributable mortality among solid organ transplant recipients in the United States: 1987 through 2014. Cancer. 2019;125(15):2647-2655. doi:10.1002/cncr.32136

70   Organ Procurement and Transplantation Network (OPTN). Living Donation. U.S. Department of Health and Human Services. https://optn.transplant.hrsa.gov/patients/about-donation/living-donation/living-donation/. Accessed July 2022.

71   Organ Procurement and Transplantation Network (OPTN). Living Donation. U.S. Department of Health and Human Services. https://optn.transplant.hrsa.gov/patients/about-donation/living-donation/living-donation/. Accessed July 2022.

72   Scientific Registry of Transplant Recipients. OPTN/SRTR 2019 Annual Data Report: Kidney. U.S. Department of Health & Human Services. https://srtr.transplant.hrsa.gov/annual_reports/2019/Kidney.aspx. Published 2019. Accessed July 2022.

73   Agrawal A, Ison M, Danziger-Isakov L. Long-Term Infectious Complications of Kidney Transplantation. *CJASN*. 2022;17(2):286-295. doi: 10.2215/CJN.15971020

74   Ojo A. Cardiovascular Complications After Renal Transplantation and Their Prevention. *Transplantation*. 2006;82(5):603-611. doi: 10.1097/01.tp.0000235527.81917.fe

75	Vella J. Kidney transplantation in adults: Risk factors for graft failure. *UpToDate.* https://www.uptodate.com/contents/kidney-transplantation-in-adults-risk-factors-for-graft-failure/print. Updated January 2023. Accessed February 2023.

76	Scientific Registry of Transplant Recipients. OPTN/SRTR 2019 Annual Data Report: Kidney. U.S. Department of Health & Human Services. https://srtr.transplant.hrsa.gov/annual_reports/2019/Kidney.aspx. Published 2019. Accessed July 2022.

77	Wang J, Skean M, Israni A. Current Status of Kidney Transplant Outcomes: Dying to Survive. *Adv Chronic Kidney Dis.* 2016;23(5):281-286

78	Hariharan S, Israni A, Danovitch, G. Long-Term Survival after Kidney Transplantation. *N Engl J Med.* 2021;385:729-743. doi: 10.1056/NEJMra2014530

79	Organ Procurement and Transplantation Network (OPTN) and Scientific Registry of Transplant Recipients. OPTN/SRTR 2017 Annual Data Report, Rockville, MD, Department of Health and Human Services. Health Resources and Services Administration, Healthcare Systems Bureau, Division of Transplantation. Published 2017. Accessed July 2022.

80	Kasiske B, Ahn Y, Conboy M, et. al. Outcomes of Living Kidney Donor Candidate Evaluations in the Living Donor Collective Pilot Registry. *Transplantation Direct.* 2021;7(5). doi: 10.1097/TXD.0000000000001143

81	Organ Procurement & Transplant Network. OPTN Policies. https://optn.transplant.hrsa.gov/media/eavh5bf3/optn_policies.pdf. Updated January 2023. Accessed September 2022.

82	Organ Procurement & Transplant Network. Guidance for the Informed Consent of Living Donors. U.S. Health and Human Services. https://optn.transplant.hrsa.gov/professionals/by-topic/guidance/guidance-for-the-informed-consent-of-living-donors/. Accessed July 2022.

83	Organ Procurement & Transplant Network. OPTN Policies. https://optn.transplant.hrsa.gov/media/eavh5bf3/optn_policies.pdf. Updated January 2023. Accessed September 2022.

84	Organ Procurement & Transplant Network. OPTN Policies. https://optn.transplant.hrsa.gov/media/eavh5bf3/optn_policies.pdf. Updated January 2023. Accessed September 2022.

85	Vella J. Kidney transplantation in adults: Risk factors for graft failure. *UpToDate.* https://www.uptodate.com/contents/kidney-transplantation-in-adults-risk-factors-for-graft-failure/print?search=living. Published July 2022. Accessed August 2022.

86	Lentine K, Smith J, Hart A, et al. OPTN/SRTR 2020 Annual Data Report: Kidney. *Am J Transplant.* 2022:21– 136. doi:10.1111/ajt.16982

87	Clayton P, McDonald S, Russ G, Chadban S. Long-Term Outcomes after Acute Rejection in Kidney Transplant Recipients: An ANZDATA Analysis. *JASN.* 2019;30 (9):1697-1707. doi: 10.1681/ASN.2018111101

88	Organ Procurement and Transplantation Network (OPTN) and Scientific Registry of Transplant Recipients. OPTN/SRTR 2011 Annual Data Report, Rockville, MD, Department of Health and Human Services, Health Resources and Services Administration, Healthcare Systems Bureau, Division of Transplantation. Published 2012. Accessed July 2022.

89 Segev D, Gentry S, Warren D, Reeb B, Montgomery R. Kidney paired donation and optimizing the use of live donor organs. *JAMA.* 2005;*293*(15): 1883–1890. doi:10.1001/jama.293.15.1883

90 Organ Procurement & Transplant Network. About CPRA. U.S. Health and Human Services. https://optn.transplant.hrsa.gov/data/allocation-calculators/about-cpra/. Accessed August 2022.

91 Veal J, Danovitch G, Nassiri N. Kidney transplantation in adults: Kidney paired donation. *UpToDate.* https://www.uptodate.com/contents/kidney-transplantation-in-adults-kidney-paired-donation. Published May 16, 2022. Accessed August 2022.

92 National Kidney Registry. Voucher Program. https://www.kidneyregistry.org/for-centers/voucher-program/. Accessed January 2023.

93 Legal Issues in Payment of Living Donors for Solid Organs. American Bar Association. https://www.americanbar.org/groups/crsj/publications/human_rights_magazine_home/human_rights_vol30_2003/spring2003/hr_spring03_livingdonors/. Published April 2003. Accessed August 2022.

94 Lentine K, Vella J. Kidney transplantation in adults: Risk of living kidney donation. *UpToDate.* https://www.uptodate.com/contents/kidney-transplantation-in-adults-risk-of-living-kidney-donation/print?search=living. Updated January 2023.

95 Jacobs C, Gross C, Messersmith E, Hong B, Gillespie B, Hill-Callahan P, et al. Emotional and Financial Experiences of Kidney Donors over the Past 50 Years: The RELIVE Study. *CJASN.* 2015;10(12):2221-223. doi: 10.2215/CJN.07120714

96 Clemens K, Boudville N, Dew M, Geddes C, Gill J, Jassal V, et al. (2011, February 22). The Long-Term Quality of Life of Living Kidney Donors: A Multicenter Cohort Study. *American Journal of Transplantation.* 2011;11(3):463-469. https://doi.org/10.1111/j.1600-6143.2010.03424.x. Accessed July 2022.

97 Lentine K, Lam N, Segev D. (2019, April 5). Risks of Living Kidney Donation. *CJASN.* 2019;14(4):597-608. doi: 10.2215/CJN.11220918

98 Gaston R, Kumar V, Matas J. Reassessing Medical Risk in Living Kidney Donors. *Journal of American Society of Nephrology.* 2015;26:1017-1019. https://www.kidneyregistry.org/wp-content/uploads/2021/03/Reassessing-Medical-Risk-in-Living-Kidney-Donors.pdf

99 Segev D, Muzaale A, Caffo B, Mehta S, Singer A, Taranto S, McBride M. et al. Perioperative Mortality and Long-term Survival Following Live Kidney Donation. *JAMA.* 2010;303(10):959-966. doi:10.1001/jama.2010.237

100 Lentine K, Vella J. Kidney transplantation in adults: Risk of living kidney donation. *UpToDate.* https://www.uptodate.com/contents/kidney-transplantation-in-adults-risk-of-living-kidney-donation/print?search=living. Updated January 2023.

101 Lentine K, Vella J. Kidney transplantation in adults: Risk of living kidney Lentine K, Vella J. Kidney transplantation in adults: Risk of living kidney donation. *UpToDate.* https://www.uptodate.com/contents/kidney-transplantation-in-adults-risk-of-living-kidney-donation/print?search=living. Updated January 2023.

102 Lentine K, Lam N, Segev D. Risks of Living Kidney Donation. *CJASN.* 2019;14(4):597-608. doi:10.2215/CJN.11220918

103   Lentine K, Vella J. Kidney transplantation in adults: Risk of living kidney donation. *UpToDate*. https://www.uptodate.com/contents/kidney-transplantation-in-adults-risk-of-living-kidney-donation/print?search=living. Updated January 2023.

104   Lentine K, Lam N, Segev D. Risks of Living Kidney Donation. *CJASN*. 2019;14(4):597-608. doi: 10.2215/CJN.11220918

105   Lentine K, Lam N, Segev D. Risks of Living Kidney Donation: Current State of Knowledge on Outcomes Important to Donors. *CJASN*. 2019;14(4):597-608. doi: 10.2215/CJN.11220918

106   Zorgdrager M, van Londen M, Westenberg L, Nieuwenhuijs-Moeke G, Lange J, et al. Chronic pain after hand-assisted laparoscopic donor nephrectomy. *Br J Surg*. 2019;106(6):711-719. doi:10.1002/bjs.11127

107   Mjoen G, Hallan S, Hartmann A, Foss A, Midtvedt K, Oyen O, et al. Long-term risks for kidney donors. *Kidney International*. 2014;86:162-167. doi: 10.1038/ki.2013.460

108   Lentine K, Vella J. Kidney transplantation in adults: Risk of living kidney donation. *UpToDate*. https://www.uptodate.com/contents/kidney-transplantation-in-adults-risk-of-living-kidney-donation/print?search=living. Updated January 2023.

109   Muzaale A, Massie A, Wang M, Montgomery R, McBride M, Wainright J, Segev, D. Risk of end-stage renal disease following live kidney donation. *JAMA*. 2014;*311*(6):579–586. doi: 10.1011/jama.2013.28514

110   Lam N, Lloyd A, Lentine K, Quinn R, Ravani P, Hemmelgarn B, et al. Changes in kidney function follow living donor nephrectomy. *Kidney International*. 2020;98(1):176-186. doi: 10.1016/j.kint.2020.03.034

111   Organ Procurement & Transplant Network. OPTN Policies. U.S. Health and Human Services. https://optn.transplant.hrsa.gov/media/eavh5bf3/optn_policies.pdf. Accessed September 2022.

112   Lam N, Lloyd A, Lentine K, Quinn R, Ravani P, Hemmelgarn B, et al. Changes in kidney function follow living donor nephrectomy. *Kidney International*. 2020 98:176-186. doi: 10.1016/j.kint.2020.03.034

113   Berglund D, Zhang L, Matas A, IbrahimH. Measrued Glomerular Filrtation Rate After Kidney Doation: No Evidence of Accelerated Decay. *Transplantation*. 2018;102(10):1756-1761. doi: 10.1097/TP.0000000000002215

114   Lentine K, Lam N, Segev D. Risks of Living Kidney Donation: Current State of Knowledge on Outcomes Important to Donors. *CJASN*. 2019;14(4):597-608. doi: 10.2215/CJN.11220918

115   Lentine K, Vella J. Kidney transplantation in adults: Risk of living kidney donation. *UpToDate*. https://www.uptodate.com/contents/kidney-transplantation-in-adults-risk-of-living-kidney-donation/print?search=living. Updated January 2023.

116   Mjoen, G., Hallan, S., Hartmann, A., Foss, A., et al. Long-term risks for kidney donors. *Kidney International*. 2014;86, 162-167.

117   Rodrigue J, Schold J, Morrissey P, Whiting J, et al. KDOC Study Group: Mood, body image, fear of kidney failure, life satisfaction, and decisional stability following living kidney donation: Findings from the KDOC study. *Am J Transplant*. 2018;18(6):1397–1407. doi: 10.1111/ajt.14618

118   Brooks, D. Clinical features, diagnosis, and prevention or incisional hernias. *UpToDate*. https://www.uptodate.com/contents/clinical-features-diagnosis-and-prevention-of-incisional-hernias. Updated July 2022. Accessed July 2022.

119   Finck D, Baumann P, Wente M, Knebel P, et al. Incisional hernia rate 3 years after midline laparotomy. *BJS*. 2013;(101)2:51–54. doi: 10.1002/bjs.9364

120   Lentine K, Vella J. Kidney transplantation in adults: Risk of living kidney donation. *UpToDate*. https://www.uptodate.com/contents/kidney-transplantation-in-adults-risk-of-living-kidney-donation/print?search=living. Updated January 2023.

121   Kasiske B, Kumar R, Kimmel P, Pesavento T, Kalil R, Kraus E, et al. Abnormalities in biomarkers of mineral and bone metabolism in kidney donors. *Kidney Int*. 2016;90(4):861-8. doi: 10.1016/j.kint.2016.05.012

122   Garg A, Nevis I, McArthur E, Sontrop J, Koval J, Ngan L, et al. Gestational Hypertension and Preeclampsia in Living Kidney Donors. *N Engl J Med*. 2015;372:14-133. doi: 10.1056/NEJMoa1408932

123   Kasiske B, Anderson-Haag T, Ibrahim H, Pesavento T, Weir M, Nogueira J, et al. A prospective controlled study of kidney donors: Baseline and 6-month follow-up. *Am J Kidney Dis*. 2013;62(3):577–586. doi: 10.1053/j.ajkd.2013.01.027

124   Rodrigue J, Fleishan A, Schold J, Morrissey P, Whiting J, Vella J. Patterns and predictors of fatigue following living donor nephrectomy: Findings from the KDOC Study. *Am J Transplant*. 2020;20(1):181-189. doi:10.111/ajt.15519

125   Garg A, Nevis I, McArthur E, Sontrop J, Koval J, Ngan L, et al. Gestational Hypertension and Preeclampsia in Living Kidney Donors. *N Engl J Med*. 2015;372:14-133. doi: 10.1056/NEJMoa1408932

126   United Network for Organ Sharing. Living Donation: Information you need to know. https://unos.org/wp-content/uploads/Brochure-107-Living-donation.pdf. Accessed January 2022.

127   National Kidney Foundation. What to Expect After Donation. https://www.kidney.org/transplantation/livingdonors/what-expect-after-donation. Accessed January 2022.

128   United Network for Organ Sharing. Living Donation: Information you need to know. https://unos.org/wp-content/uploads/Brochure-107-Living-donation.pdf. Accessed January 2022.

129   Lam N, Garg A, Segev D, et al. Gout after living kidney donation: correlations with demographic traits and renal complications. *Am J Nephrol*. 2015;41(3):231-240. doi:10.1159/000381291

130   Pain Medicines (Analgesics). National Kidney Foundation. https://www.kidney.org/atoz/content/painmeds_analgesics. Accessed February 2022.

131   Lentine K, Vella J. Kidney transplantation in adults: Risk of living kidney donation. *UpToDate*. https://www.uptodate.com/contents/kidney-transplantation-in-adults-risk-of-living-kidney-donation/print?search=living. Updated January 2023.

132   Nanidis T, Antcliffe D, Kokkinos C, Borysiewicz C, Darzi A, Tekkis P, et al. Laparoscopic versus open live donor nephrectomy in renal transplantation: a meta-analysis. *Annals of Surgery*. 2008;247(1):58–70. doi:10.1097/SLA.0b0

133   MedlinePlus. Kidney Removal. National Library of Medicine. https://medlineplus.gov/ency/article/003001.htm. Accessed August 2022.

135   Garg A, Nevis I, McArthur E, Sontrop J, Koval J, Ngan L, et al. Gestational Hypertension and Preeclampsia in Living Kidney Donors. *N Engl J Med*. 2015;372:14-133. doi: 10.1056/NEJMoa1408932

136   What to Expect After Donation. National Kidney Foundation. https://www.kidney.org/transplantation/livingdonors/what-expect-after-donation. Accessed February 2022.

137   United Network for Organ Sharing. Living Donation: Information you need to know. https://unos.org/wp-content/uploads/Brochure-107-Living-donation.pdf. Accessed January 2022.

138   Lentine K, Vella J. Kidney transplantation in adults: Risk of living kidney donation. *UpToDate*. https://www.uptodate.com/contents/kidney-transplantation-in-adults-risk-of-living-kidney-donation/print?search=living. Updated January 2023.

139   American Transplant Foundation. Living Donor Laws: State by State and Federal. https://www.americantransplantfoundation.org/wp-content/uploads/2020/03/Living_Donor_Laws_Federal_And_State_By_State.pdf. Published March 2020. Accessed January 2023.

140   Making the Decision to Donate. National Kidney Foundation. https://www.kidney.org/transplantation/livingdonors/making-decision-to-donate. Accessed August 2022.

141   Rodrigue J, Schold J, Morrissey P, Whiting J, et al. KDOC Study Group: Mood, body image, fear of kidney failure, life satisfaction, and decisional stability following living kidney donation: Findings from the KDOC study. *Am J Transplant*. 2018;18(6):1397–1407. doi: 10.1111/ajt.14618

142   Clemens K, Boudville N, Dew M, Gill J, Jassal V, Klarenback S, et al. The Long-Term Quality of Life of Living Kidney Donors: A Multicenter Cohort Study. *Am J Transplant*. 2011;11(3):463-469. doi: 10.1111/j.1600-6143.2010.03424.x

143   Jacobs C, Gross C, Messersmith E, Hong B, Gillespie B, Hill-Callahan, et al. Emotional and Financial Experiences of Kidney Donors over the Past 50 Years: The RELIVE Study. *CJASN*, 2015;10(12):2221-223. doi: 10.2215/CJN.07120714

144   Clemens K, Boudville N, Dew M, Gill J, Jassal V, Klarenback S, et al. The Long-Term Quality of Life of Living Kidney Donors: A Multicenter Cohort Study. *Am J Transplant*. 2011;11(3):463-469. doi: 10.1111/j.1600-6143.2010.03424.x

145   Lentine K, Lam N, Segev D. Risks of Living Kidney Donation. *CJASN*. 2019;14(4):597-608. doi: 10.2215/CJN.11220918

146   Post S. Altruism, happiness, and health: it's good to be good. *Int J Behav Med*. 2005;12:66–77. doi: 10.1207/s15327558ijbm1202_4

147   Healy K. How Giving Keeps on Giving. Stanford Social Innovation Review. https://ssir.org/books/reviews/entry/how_giving_keeps_on_giving#. Published Winter 2015. Accessed November 2022.

148   Lawton R, Gramatki I, Watt W, Fujiwara D. Does Volunteering Make Us Happier, or Are Happier People More Likely to Volunteer? Addressing the Problem of Reverse Causality When Estimating the Wellbeing Impacts of Volunteering. *J Happiness Stud*. 2021;22:599-624. doi: 0.1007/s10902-020-00242-8

149 Stanford Medicine Children's Health. Living donor transplantation has emotional benefits, too. https://healthier.stanfordchildrens.org/en/living-donor-transplantation-emotional-benefits/. Published March 2014. Accessed July 2022.

150 Van Pilsum Rasmussen S, Robin M, Saha A, Eno A. The Tangible Benefits of Living Donation: Results of a Qualitative Study of Living Kidney Donors. *Transplant Direct.* 2020;6(12):e626. doi: 10.1097/TXD.0000000000001068

151 Van Pilsum Rasmussen S, Robin M, Saha A, Eno A. The Tangible Benefits of Living Donation: Results of a Qualitative Study of Living Kidney Donors. *Transplant Direct.* 2020;6(12):e626. doi: 10.1097/TXD.0000000000001068

152 Holscher C, Leanza J, Thomas A, Waldram M, Haugen C, Jackson K, et al. Anxiety, depression, and regret of donation in living kidney donors. *BMC Nephrol.* 2018;19(218). doi: 10.1186/s12882-018-1024-0

153 Rodrigue J, Schold J, Morrissey P, Whiting J, et al. KDOC Study Group: Mood, body image, fear of kidney failure, life satisfaction, and decisional stability following living kidney donation: Findings from the KDOC study. *Am J Transplant.* 2018;18(6):1397–1407. doi: 10.1111/ajt.14618

154 Rodrigue J, Schold J, Morrissey P, Whiting J, et al. KDOC Study Group: Mood, body image, fear of kidney failure, life satisfaction, and decisional stability following living kidney donation: Findings from the KDOC study. *Am J Transplant.* 2018;18(6):1397–1407. doi: 10.1111/ajt.14618

155 Lentine K, Schnitzler M, Xiao H, Axelrod D, Davis C, McCabe M, et al. Depression diagnoses after living kidney donation: linking U.S. Registry data and administrative claims. *Transplantation.* 2014;94(1):7–83. doi: 10.1097/TP.0b013e318253f1bc

156 Jowsey S, Jacobs C, Hong B, Messersmith E, Gillespie B, Beebe T, et al. Emotional Well-Being of Living Kidney Donors: Findings From the RELIVE Study. *Am J Transplant.* 2014;14(11):2535-2544. doi:10.1111/ajt.12906

157 Lentine K, Lam N, Segev D. Risks of Living Kidney Donation. *CJASN.* 2019;14(4):597-608. doi: 10.2215/CJN.11220918

158 Rodrigue J, Schold J, Morrissey P, Whiting J, et al. KDOC Study Group: Mood, body image, fear of kidney failure, life satisfaction, and decisional stability following living kidney donation: Findings from the KDOC study. *Am J Transplant.* 2018;18(6):1397–1407. doi: 10.1111/ajt.14618

159 Organ Procurement & Transplantation Network. Guidance for the Development of Program-Specific Living Kidney Donor Medical Evaluation Protocols. U.S. Department of Health & Human Services. https://optn.transplant.hrsa.gov/professionals/by-topic/guidance/guidance-for-the-development-of-program-specific-living-kidney-donor-medical-evaluation-protocols/. Accessed August 2022.

160 Levey A, Inker L. GFR Evaluation in Living Kidney Donor Candidates. *J Am Soc Nephrol.* 2017;28(4):1062-1071. doi: 10.1681/ASN.2016070790

161 Rastogi A. Kidney Disease: What You Should Know. YouTube. https://www.youtube.com/watch?v=W0OmgjNRSIE. Published August 2018.

162 Benefits of Physical Activity. National Institute of Diabetes and Digestive and Kid-

ney Diseases. Managing Chronic Kidney Disease. https://www.niddk.nih.gov/health-information/kidney-disease/chronic-kidney-disease-ckd/managing#becareful. Updated October 2016. Accessed May 2022.

163 Centers for Disease Control and Prevention. https://www.cdc.gov/physicalactivity/basics/pa-health/index.htm. Updated June 2022. Accessed June 2022.

164 Mustian M, Hanaway M, Kumar V, Reed R, Shelton B, Grant R, et al. Patient Perspectives on Weight Management for Living Kidney Donation. *J Surg Res*. 2019;244:50–56. doi: 10.1016/j.jss.2019.06.026

165 Bugeja A, Harris S, Ernst J, Burns K, Knoll G. Changes in Body Weight Before and After Kidney Donation. *Can J Kidney Health Dis*. 2019. doi: 10.1177/2054358119847203

166 The Surprising Link Between Chronic Kidney Disease, Diabetes, and Heart Disease. Centers for Disease Control and Prevention. https://www.cdc.gov/kidneydisease/publications-resources/link-between-ckd-diabetes-heart-disease.html. Updated July 2022. Accessed August 2022.

167 High Blood Pressure & Kidney Disease. National Institutes of Health. https://www.niddk.nih.gov/health-information/kidney-disease/high-blood-pressure. Updated March 2022. Accessed August 2022.

168 Rastogi A. Kidney Disease: What You Should Know. YouTube. https://www.youtube.com/watch?v=W0OmgjNRSIE. Published August 2018.

169 Salt and Sodium. Harvard T.H. Chan School of Public Health. https://www.hsph.harvard.edu/nutritionsource/salt-and-sodium/. Accessed August 2022.

170 Choose Heart-Healthy Foods. National Heart, Lung, and Blood Institute. https://www.nhlbi.nih.gov/health/heart-healthy-living/healthy-foods. Updated March 2022. Accessed August 2022.

171 Getting Active to Control High Blood Pressure. American Heart Association. https://www.heart.org/en/health-topics/high-blood-pressure/changes-you-can-make-to-manage-high-blood-pressure/getting-active-to-control-high-blood-pressure. Published October 2016. Accessed August 2022.

172 Pahwa R, Goyal A, Jialal I. Chronic Inflammation. https://www.ncbi.nlm.nih.gov/books/NBK493173/. Updated August 2022. Accessed August 2022.

173 Ko G, Rhee C, Kalantar-Zadeh K, Joshi S. The Effects of High-Protein Diets on Kidney Health and Longevity. *JASN*. 2020;31(8):1667–1679. doi: 10.1681/ASN.2020010028

174 Delimaris I. Adverse Effects Associated with Protein Intake above the Recommended Dietary Allowance for Adults. *ISRN nutrition*. 2013;126929. doi: 10.5402/2013/126929

175 Ko G, Obi Y, Tortorici A, Kalantar-Zadeh K. Dietary protein intake and chronic kidney disease. *Curr Opin Clin Nutr Metab Care*. 2017;20(1):77–85. doi: 10.1097/MCO.0000000000000342

176 Greger, M. The Effect of Animal Protein on the Kidneys. NutritionFacts.org. https://nutritionfacts.org/2018/02/08/the-effect-of-animal-protein-on-the-kidneys/. Published February 2018. Accessed July 2022.

178 Trevisan R, Nosadini R, Fioretto P, Borsato M, Sacerdoti D, Viberti G. Renal metabolic and hormonal responses to ingestion of animal and vegetable proteins. *Kidney Int*. 1990;38(1):136–144. doi: 10.1038/ki.1990.178

179   Joshi S, Shah S, Kalantar-Zadeh K. Adequacy of Plant-Based Proteins in Chronic Kidney Disease. *J Ren Nutr.* 2019;29(2):112-117. doi: 10.1053/j.jrn.2018.06.006

180   Joshi S, Shah S, Kalantar-Zadeh K. Adequacy of Plant-Based Proteins in Chronic Kidney Disease. *J Ren Nutr.* 2019;29(2):112-117. doi: 10.1053/j.jrn.2018.06.006

181   Diabetes and. Chronic Kidney Disease. Centers for Disease Control and Prevention. https://www.cdc.gov/diabetes/managing/diabetes-kidney-disease.html. Updated May 2021.Accessed August 2022.

182   Diabetes Statistics. National Institute of Diabetes and Digestive and Kidney Diseases. https://www.niddk.nih.gov/health-information/health-statistics/diabetes-statistics. Updated May 2018. Accessed August 2022.

183   Insulin Resistance & Prediabetes. National Institute of Diabetes and Digestive and Kidney Diseases. https://www.niddk.nih.gov/health-information/diabetes/overview/what-is-diabetes/prediabetes-insulin-resistance. Updated December 2020. Accessed August 2022.

184   MedlinePlus. Blood Sugar. National Library of Medicine. https://medlineplus.gov/bloodsugar.html. Updated June 2017. Accessed August 2022.

185   All About Your A1C. Centers for Disease Control and Prevention. https://www.cdc.gov/diabetes/managing/managing-blood-sugar/a1c.html. Updated August 10, 2021. Accessed August 2022.

186   All About Your A1C. Centers for Disease Control and Prevention. https://www.cdc.gov/diabetes/managing/managing-blood-sugar/a1c.html. Updated August 10, 2021. Accessed August 2022.

187   Insulin Resistance & Prediabetes. National Institute of Diabetes and Digestive and Kidney Diseases. https://www.niddk.nih.gov/health-information/diabetes/overview/what-is-diabetes/prediabetes-insulin-resistance. Updated December 2020. Accessed August 2022.

188   Fiber. Harvard T.H. Chan School of Public Health. https://www.hsph.harvard.edu/nutritionsource/carbohydrates/fiber/. Accessed August 2022.

189   Carbohydrates and Blood Sugar. Harvard T.H. Chan School of Public Health. https://www.hsph.harvard.edu/nutritionsource/carbohydrates/carbohydrates-and-blood-sugar/#ref13. Accessed August 2022.

190   Livesey G, Taylor R, Livesey H, Liu S. Is there a dose-response relation of dietary glycemic load to risk of type 2 diabetes? Meta-analysis of prospective cohort studies. *Am J Clin Nutr.* 2013;97:584-96. doi: 10.3945/ajcn.112.041467

191   Grady D. Drinking More Water for Prevention of Recurrent Cystitis. *JAMA Intern Med.* 2018;178(11):1515. doi:10.1001/jamainternmed.2018.4195

192   Can Dehydration Affect Your Kidneys? National Kidney Foundation. https://www.kidney.org/newsletter/can-dehydration-affect-your-kidneys. Accessed April 2022.

193   MedlinePlus. Dehydration. National Library of Medicine. https://medlineplus.gov/dehydration.html. Updated May 2019. Accessed April 2022.

194   Tips for drinking more water. Mayo Clinic Health Systems. https://www.mayoclinichealthsystem.org/hometown-health/speaking-of-health/tips-for-drinking-more-water. Updated July 2021. Accessed April 2022.

195 Reports Set Dietary Intake Levels for Water, Salt, and Potassium To Maintain Health and Reduce Chronic Disease Risk. National Academies of Sciences, Engineering, Medicine. https://www.nationalacademies.org/news/2004/02/report-sets-dietary-intake-levels-for-water-salt-and-potassium-to-maintain-health-and-reduce-chronic-disease-risk. Published February 2004. Accessed April 2022.

196 Alcohol and Your Kidneys. National Kidney Foundation. https://www.kidney.org/atoz/content/alcohol. Accessed April 2022.

197 Limiting Alcohol to Manage High Blood Pressure. American Heart Association. (2016, October 31). https://www.heart.org/en/health-topics/high-blood-pressure/changes-you-can-make-to-manage-high-blood-pressure/limiting-alcohol-to-manage-high-blood-pressure. Published October 2016. Accessed May 2022.

198 Can Dehydration Affect Your Kidneys? National Kidney Foundation. https://www.kidney.org/newsletter/can-dehydration-affect-your-kidneys. Accessed April 2022.

199 Preventing Chronic Kidney Disease. National Institute of Diabetes and Digestive and Kidney Diseases. https://www.niddk.nih.gov/health-information/kidney-disease/chronic-kidney-disease-ckd/prevention. Updated October 2016. Accessed April 2022.

200 Alcohol and Your Kidneys. National Kidney Foundation. https://www.kidney.org/atoz/content/alcohol. Accessed April 2022.

201 How much physical activity do adults need? Centers for Disease Control and Prevention. https://www.cdc.gov/physicalactivity/basics/adults/index.htm. Updated 2022. Accessed June 2022.

202 Which Drugs are Harmful to Your Kidneys? National Kidney Foundation. https://www.kidney.org/atoz/content/drugs-your-kidneys. Accessed February 2022.

203 Pain Medicines (Analgesics). National Kidney Foundation. https://www.kidney.org/atoz/content/painmeds_analgesics. Accessed February 2022.

204 Medline Plus. Over-the-counter pain relievers. National Library of Medicine. https://medlineplus.gov/ency/article/002123.htm. Accessed February 2022.

205 Pain Medicines (Analgesics). National Kidney Foundation. https://www.kidney.org/atoz/content/painmeds_analgesics. Accessed February 2022.

206 Pain Medicines (Analgesics). National Kidney Foundation. https://www.kidney.org/atoz/content/painmeds_analgesics. Accessed February 2022.

207 Richardson M, Nolin T. A Decade After the KDOQI CKD Guidelines: Impact on Medication Safety. *AJKD*. 2012;60(5):713-715 doi: 10.1053/j.ajkd.2012.08.018

208 Izzedine H, Launay-Vacher V, Deray G. Antiviral Drug-Induced Nephrotoxicity. *AJKD*. 2005;45(5):804-817 doi: 10.1053/j.ajkd.2005.02.010

209 5 Drugs You May Need to Avoid or Adjust if You Have Kidney Disease. National Kidney Foundation. https://www.kidney.org/atoz/content/5-drugs-you-may-need-to-avoid-or-adjust-if-you-have-kidney-disease. Accessed March 2022.

210 Contrast Dye and the Kidneys. National Kidney Foundation. https://www.kidney.org/atoz/content/Contrast-Dye-and-Kidneys. Accessed March 2022.

211 Oral Sodium Phosphate Safety. National Kidney Foundation. https://www.kidney.org/atoz/content/oralsodium. Accessed March 2022.

212   Lee J, Keum B, Yoo I, Kim S, Choi H, Kim E, et al. Polyethylene glycol plus ascorbic acid for bowel preparation in chronic kidney disease. *Medicine*. 2016;95(36):e4755. doi: 10.1097/MD.0000000000004755

213   Herbal Supplements and Kidney Disease. National Kidney Foundation. https://www.kidney.org/atoz/content/herbalsupp. Accessed April 2022.

214   Leonberg-Yoo A, Johnson D, Persun N, Bahrainwala J, Reese P, Naji A. Use of Dietary Supplements in Living Kidney Donors: A Critical Review. Am J Kidney Diseases. 2020;76(6):851-860 doi:10.1053/j.ajkd.2020.03.030

215   Singh V, Singh N, Jaggi A. A review on renal toxicity profile of common abusive drugs. *Korean J. Physiol. Pharmacol.* 2013;17(4): 347–357. doi: 10.4196/kjpp.2013.17.4.347

216   Which Drugs are Harmful to Your Kidneys? National Kidney Foundation. https://www.kidney.org/atoz/content/drugs-your-kidneys. Accessed April 2022.

217   Rein J, Texter L, Wurfel M, Siew E, Garg A, Tan T, Kimmel P, et al. Marijuana Use and Kidney Outcomes in the ASSESS-ALI Cohort. JASN: Kidney Week 2018. https://www.asn-online.org/education/kidneyweek/archives/KW18Abstracts.pdf. Published 2018. Accessed January 2023.

218   Ishida J, Auer R, Vittinghoff E, Plethcer M, Reis J, Sidney S, et al. Marijuana Use and Estimated Glomerular Filtration Rate in Young Adults. *CJASN*. 2017;12(10):1578-1587. doi: 10.2215/CJN.01530217

219   Health Effects of Smoking & Tobacco Use. Centers for Disease Control and Prevention. https://www.cdc.gov/tobacco/basic_information/health_effects/index.htm. Updated April 2020. Accessed April 2022.

220   Health Effects of Cigarette Smoking. Centers for Disease Control and Prevention. https://www.cdc.gov/tobacco/data_statistics/fact_sheets/health_effects/effects_cig_smoking/index.htm. Updated October 2021. Accessed April 2022.

221   Stress and Your Kidneys. National Kidney Foundation. https://www.kidney.org/atoz/content/Stress_and_your_Kidneys. Accessed May 2022.

222   Understanding the stress response. Harvard Health Publishing. (2020, July 06). https://www.health.harvard.edu/staying-healthy/understanding-the-stress-response. Published July 2020. Accessed May 2022.

223   Stress and Your Kidneys. National Kidney Foundation. https://www.kidney.org/atoz/content/Stress_and_your_Kidneys. Accessed May 2022.

By Living Kidney Donors

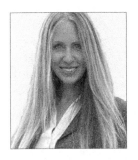

Tami Winchell, BCPA is a Board-Certified Patient Advocate, health writer, and nutritionist focused on the improvement of health and well-being through education and mentorship. Her commitment to improved healthcare outcomes and accessibility is evident in her work with esteemed organizations such as UCLA Health, the National Patient Advocacy Foundation, the National Kidney Foundation, and the PKD Foundation. In 2014, she donated a kidney to her husband after his kidneys failed due to polycystic kidney disease. Since then, she has been a loyal mentor for living kidney donors and transplant recipients, helping them navigate their transplant journeys and encouraging responsible, informed living kidney donation.

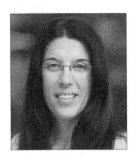

Laura Perin, Ph.D. is an Associate Professor and co-Director of the GOFARR laboratory, an NIH-funded research laboratory. Dr. Perin obtained a master's degree in Biological Sciences at the University of Padova, Italy, and a Ph.D. through a joint Ph.D. program between the Harvard Medical School, Boston, and the University of Padova, Italy. Dr. Perin's research focuses on understanding the molecular mechanisms that regulate kidney disease and pediatric kidney cancer. Dr. Perin published more than 60 peer-reviewed publications on kidney disease and volunteers on various committees and foundations. Dr. Perin is dedicated to finding new therapeutic approaches for patients suffering from progressive renal disease. Dr. Perin is also a living kidney donor; she donated a kidney to her husband affected by polycystic kidney disease in 2021 and since has been highly involved in advocating responsible living kidney donation.

Made in the USA
Las Vegas, NV
28 September 2023

78279858R00095